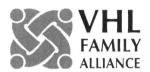

The VHL Handbook

What you Need to Know about VHL

*A Reference Handbook
for people with von Hippel-Lindau,
their families, and support personnel*

Fourth edition, Revised 2012
ISBN 978-147500-75-96

*Copyright 1993, 1997, 1999. 2005, 2012 VHL Family Alliance
All rights reserved.*
International edition (English) ISBN 978-147500-75-96

French edition ISBN 1-929539-06-1
Spanish edition ISBN 1-929539-07-X
Japanese edition ISBN 1-929539-08-8
Chinese edition ISBN 1-929539-09-6
Dutch edition ISBN 1-929539-10-X
Italian edition ISBN 1-929539-11-8
Arabic edition, ISBN 1-929539-16-9
Hindi edition, ISBN 1-929539-05-3

Available in additional languages on request.

DISCLAIMER

This book is intended to add to, not replace, conversations between a patient and a physician, as the specific details and the patient's total health situation needs to be considered in making the final decisions about treatment. The content of the book should not be taken nor relied upon as medical advice on how to treat your specific manifestation of this condition. Rather, by providing context and understanding, we hope that this book will empower the patient to be a better partner in his or her own care, and will facilitate constructive conversations between patient and physician.

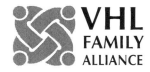

Dedicated to improving diagnosis, treatment, and quality of life for individuals and families affected by VHL

2001 Beacon Street, Suite 208, Boston, MA 02135-7787 USA
+1-617-277-5667, (800) 767-4VHL
Fax: +1-858-712-8712; E-mail: info@vhl.org
http://www.vhl.org
http://www.vhl-europa.org

VHL Family Alliance

The VHL Family Alliance was founded in 1993 as a partnership among people affected by von Hippel-Lindau disease, interested health care professionals and researchers in the field. Partnership in the Alliance includes the newsletter (3-4 issues a year), and one copy of all publications.

The Alliance is supported by the generosity of its partners and supporters.

Caring...
an international network of family support groups
  Sharing...
  in person, on the telephone hotline, on the internet, and through the *VHL Family Forum*
    Learning...
    from each other and from our physicians and medical teams
      Educating...
      ourselves, the medical community, and the general public
        Funding...
        better ways of managing VHL and similar tumor conditions for everyone.
          Research...
          working for a cure through tissue banking, data collection, and awarding grants.

Clinical Care Centers. Call or see http://vhl.org/ccc for referral to an institution participating in the VHLFA information network.

Local Family Support Chapters. Call for the contact person in your area, or to start a new group. Support communities also exist on the internet in many languages, including English, Spanish, German, French, Italian, and Japanese.

Preface

VHL FAMILY ALLIANCE

This information has been compiled to help individuals with VHL, their families, and other interested people understand VHL. The information presented here is intended to add to conversations with physicians and other health care providers. No brochure can replace personal conversations and personal advice about questions on treatment.

One of our primary goals is to give affected individuals and their families greater confidence in the future. With early detection and appropriate treatment, there is more hope today for families with von Hippel-Lindau disease than ever before. Recent research on VHL and related diseases has led to better methods of diagnosis and treatment. Knowledge is increasing rapidly by the open sharing of information throughout the world among families, health professionals and the research community.

We acknowledge the important contributions to this booklet of our many collaborators and reviewers, both family members and physicians. Knowledge and effective treatment of VHL has been accelerated since 1993 through international cooperation, fostered in particular by symposia:

- Freiburg, Germany, 1994, led by Dr. Hartmut Neumann
- Honolulu, Hawaii, USA, 1996, led by Drs. Y. Edward Hsia, Berton Zbar, and J. M. Lamiell
- Paris, France, 1998, led by Dr. Stéphane Richard
- Rochester, Minnesota, USA, 2000, led by Dr. Virginia Michels
- Padua, Italy, 2002, led by Dr. Giuseppe Opocher
- Kochi, Japan, 2004, led by Dr. Taro Shuin
- London, Ontario, Canada, 2006, led by Dr. Stephen Pautler
- Roskilde, Denmark, 2008, led by Dr. Marie Luise Bisgaard
- Rio de Janeiro, Brazil, 2010, led by Dr. Jose Claudio Casali da Rocha
- Houston, Texas, 2012, led by Dr. Eric Jonasch

and by several extensive research projects—in the United States under Drs. W. Marston Linehan, Edward H. Oldfield, and Russell R. Lonser; in England under Dr. Eamonn Maher; in France under Dr. Stéphane Richard; in Germany under Dr. Hartmut Neumann; and in Japan under Dr. Taro Shuin. Local language editions have been prepared and are being updated by a number of our country affiliates worldwide.

Revision 4, 2012, updates the clinical information throughout, reflecting the many advances in screening, diagnosis, treatment, and quality of life. It is clear that the best way to manage VHL is to identify issues early, monitor and treat them appropriately with minimal invasion and damage, and focus on long-term health. The VHL Family Alliance looks forward to working with you and your medical team.

This book is available in print or electronic version from major book sellers worldwide.

This text is also available over the Internet, both as a Web service and for download as pdf or e-book.
See www.vhl.org.

Please note that the *VHL Handbook Kids' Edition*, specifically geared toward children and their families, is also available in multiple languages in print, e-book, or pdf.

Throughout this booklet, words that may be new to readers are printed for the first time in italics. Definitions of these and other medical terms related to VHL appear at the back of this booklet. A "sounds-like" spelling is also given for some words.

Suggestions and comments to make future editions of this booklet even better are always welcome

— *Joyce Wilcox Graff, Editor, VHL Family Alliance, January 2012*

Table of Contents

Preface 5

What is VHL? 11
- Angiomas, Hemangioblastomas,
  Cysts and Tumors 12
- What is Cancer? 14
- How Do People get VHL? 15
- Early Detection 16
- General Recommendations for Screening 18

Possible Manifestations 21
- VHL in the Retina 21
- VHL in the Brain and Spinal Cord 23
- Considering Stereotactic Radiosurgery 25
- Hearing Changes and VHL 29
- VHL and Your Reproductive Health 31
  - *For Men* 32
  - *For Women* 35
- Pregnancy and VHL 36
- Pre-Implantation Genetic Diagnosis 38
- Blood Pressure, Emotions, and VHL 40
- VHL in the Kidneys 44
- VHL in the Pancreas 48

Diagnosis, Treatment, and Research 53
- Diagnosis and Treatment 53
- Genetic Research and VHL 54
- Progress Toward a Cure 57
- Promoting Research and Clinical Trials 63

Living Well with VHL 65
- The Healthy Eating Plate 68
- Living with Knowing 70
- Family Support 73
- Talking with Children about VHL 74
- Some Suggestions for Reading 75
- Questions to Ask the Doctor 75
- The VHL Athlete 77
- Reminder Calendar 78

Suggested Screening Guidelines 79
- Commonly Occurring VHL Manifestations 82
- Common Treatment Recommendations 84

    Preparing for Pheo Testing 86
        Preparation for Blood Testing 87
        Preparation for 24-hour Urine Testing 88

Obtaining DNA Testing **91**

Medical Terms **95**

Prepared by **107**

Tissue Bank **111**
    Donor Registration Form. 113
    Brief Medical History for the Tissue Bank .114

Keeping Current **115**
    Support our Efforts! 117

List of Figures

Figure 1: Principal lesions of VHL and their frequency 13

Figure 2: Inheritance of a dominant gene 15

Figure 3: Ultrasound scanning. 19

Figure 4: Ophthalmologist. 22

Figure 5: The inner ear, showing the endolymphatic sac (ELS). . .30

Figure 6: Epididymis 33

Figure 7: Broad ligament 35

Figure 8: Kidney, pancreas, and adrenal glands 40

Figure 9: Dandelions. 51

Figure 10: VHL gene location 55

Figure 11: Path to development of a tumor. 56

Figure 12: Black box 58

Figure 13: The VHL complex. 59

Figure 14: Pathways in the cell 60

Figure 15: The Genetics of kidney cancer 62

Figure 16: Healthy Eating Plate. 66

Figure 17: The Art of Conscious Living. 71

Figure 18: "Self-help is barn raising revisited." 73

List of Tables

Table 1: Assessing the risk level of a pancreatic neuroendocrine tumor 51

Table 2: Genotype-phenotype classifications 61

Table 3: Occurrence and age of onset in VHL..................83

> Friendship is born at that moment when
> one person says to another,
> "What! You too?
> I thought I was the only one."
> — C. S. Lewis

Section 1:
What is VHL? ...

Von Hippel-Lindau, abbreviated VHL, is one of more than 7000 known inherited disorders. *Tumors* will develop in one or more parts of the body. Many of these tumors involve the abnormal growth of blood vessels in different organs of the body.

While blood vessels normally branch out like trees, in people with VHL little knots of blood *capillaries* sometimes occur in the brain, spinal cord, or retina. These little knots are called *angiomas*, or *hemangioblastomas*. In other parts of the body the tumors of VHL are called by other names.

These tumors themselves may cause problems, or problems may develop around them. For this reason they need to be carefully monitored by your medical team.

VHL is different in every patient. Even in the same family, people may show only one or several features of VHL. Since it is impossible to predict exactly which one or more manifestations of VHL each person will have, it is important to continue to check for all the possibilities throughout a person's lifetime.

Dr. Eugen von Hippel, a German *ophthalmologist*, described the angiomas in the eye in 1893–1911. His name was originally used only in association with VHL in the *retina*.

Dr. Arvid Lindau, a Swedish pathologist, first described the angiomas of the *cerebellum* and spine in 1926. His description included a systematic compilation of all other published patients, including those of von Hippel, and described changes in different abdominal organs. We now understand that both these physicians were describing different aspects of the same disease.

Von Hippel-Lindau (VHL) is different from most other conditions in that it has no single primary *symptom*, that it does not occur exclusively in one organ of the body, and that it does not always occur in a particular age group. The condition is hereditary, but the health problems of the involved families and the specialties of the attending physicians are so varied that the common cause may not be recognized for many years. In addition, the appearance and severity of the condition are so variable that many members of the family may have only some relatively harmless issue, while others may have a serious illness.

With careful *monitoring*, early detection, and appropriate treatment, the most harmful consequences of this *gene* can be greatly reduced, or in some cases even prevented entirely.

Researchers are also finding that a significant number of new cases are occurring. As many as 20 percent of the families seen at centers around the world are the first in their family ever to have VHL. We do not yet understand why this is happening, but it underscores the importance of the need for careful *differential diagnosis* in all people, not just those in families known to be at risk for VHL.

Angiomas, Hemangioblastomas, Cysts and Tumors

Angiomas may occur in several parts of the body. Angiomas in the brain or spinal cord are called *hemangioblastomas*. The pressure they exert may in itself cause symptoms. They may press on nerve or brain tissue and cause symptoms such as headaches, problems with balance when walking, or weakness of arms and legs.

If the angioma grows, the walls of the blood vessels may weaken and some blood leakage may occur, causing damage to surrounding tissues. Blood or fluid leakage from angiomas in the retina, for example, can interfere with vision. Early detection, careful monitoring of the eye, and treatment when needed are very important to maintain healthy vision.

Cysts may grow up around angiomas. Cysts are fluid-filled sacs which may exert pressure or create blockages that can cause symptoms.

Some male patients experience tumors in the scrotal sacs. These tumors are almost always *benign*, but should be

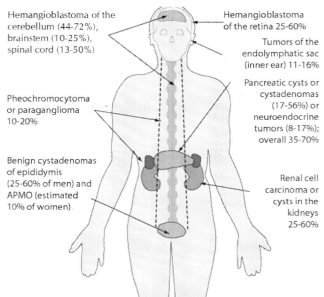

Figure 1: Principal lesions of VHL and their frequency. People with VHL will usually experience one or more of the tumors shown. Frequency varies in different families, and statistics from particular countries may differ widely for this reason. French families are more likely to have CNS lesions, German families are more likely to have pheochromocytomas, and Japanese families are more likely to have kidney tumors. The ranges shown here were compiled by the U.S. National Institutes of Health from a large international pool of patients. Figure based on an illustration from the U.S. NIH. Data from Lonser et al., *Lancet* 2003, 361: 2059-67, and *N. E. J. Med.* 2004 350:2481-2486 and G. P. James, Hastening the Road to Diagnosis, re APMO.

examined by your *urologist*. Similarly, women may have benign cysts and tumors among the reproductive organs, which need careful monitoring.

Cysts and tumors may occur in the *kidney*, *pancreas*, and *adrenal glands*. These cysts frequently cause no symptoms, but must be monitored for changes. Early *signs* of adrenal tumors may be high blood pressure, panic attacks, or heavy sweating. Early signs of pancreatic cysts and tumors may be digestive complaints like bloating or disturbance of bowel and bladder function. Some of these tumors are benign, while others are cancerous. Early detection and careful monitoring are particularly important for these organ systems, usually with yearly *MRI*, assisted by CT or *ultrasound* scanning. (See Figure 1.)

What is Cancer?

Cancer can be a frightening word. Families need to know that cancer can occur with VHL. However, with careful early monitoring and treatment, the worst possibilities of cancer may never occur.

Cancer is not one disease, it is a group of more than 100 different diseases. While each cancer differs from the others in many ways, every cancer is a disease of some of the body's cells. Cancer associated with VHL is limited to specific types.

Healthy cells that make up the body's tissues grow, divide, and replace themselves in an orderly way. This process keeps the body in good repair. Sometimes, however, normal cells lose their ability to limit and direct their growth. They divide too rapidly and grow without any order. Too much tissue is produced, and tumors begin to form. Tumors can be benign or *malignant*.

- Benign tumors are not cancerous and do not spread. VHL tumors of the brain, spinal cord, and retina are benign.
- Malignant tumors are cancerous. They can invade and destroy nearby healthy tissues and organs. Cancer cells can also spread, or metastasize, to other parts of the body and form new tumors. VHL tumors in the kidney and pancreas may become malignant.

Because VHL can cause malignant tumors in the *visceral* organ systems, it is considered one of a group of *familial* cancer risk factors, which are transmitted genetically. The objective is to find tumors early, watch for signs that a tumor is becoming aggressive in its behavior, and to remove or disable the tumor before it invades other tissues. Since these tumors are inside the body, medical imaging techniques are needed to find and watch them.

Not all tumors require surgery when they are found. Research is ongoing to learn more about how to tell when a tumor is getting worrisome and requires action. You and your family can help researchers learn more about how long we can safely watch tumors by sharing your family's own experiences. Please contact the VHL Family Alliance for more information on researching your family tree.

How Do People get VHL?

Von Hippel-Lindau is caused by an alteration in one of your two copies of a gene referred to as the VHL gene. This altered gene may be transmitted genetically, following a dominant pattern of inheritance. Each child receives one gene of each pair from each parent. If one parent has an alteration (*mutation*) in a dominant gene, each child has a fifty-fifty chance of inheriting that gene. One copy of the altered gene is sufficient to produce the disease. VHL is sometimes referred to as an *autosomal* dominant trait, meaning that it is not limited to one sex, but may occur in both men and women. (See Figure 2.)

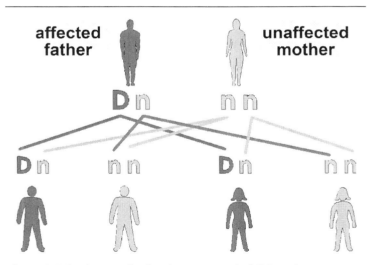

Figure 2: Inheritance of a dominant gene. A child receives one gene in each pair from each parent. If one parent has a Dominant gene (D), each child has a fifty-fifty chance of inheriting the condition. Dominant genes dominate their normal counterparts (n). A dominant gene can be inherited by either a male or female child, from an affected mother or father. *Illustration from the March of Dimes.*

Anyone with a parent with VHL and most people with a brother or sister with VHL is at 50 percent risk of having VHL. Anyone with an aunt, uncle, cousin, or grandparent with VHL may also be at risk. The only way to determine for sure that someone does not have an altered VHL gene is through DNA testing. (See Section 6, *Obtaining DNA Testing*.) Even in people who have an alteration in the VHL gene there is a wide variation in the age at which angiomas and other VHL tumors begin to grow, the organ system in which they grow, and the severity of the involvement. Every person is different.

The booklet *Your Family Health Tree*, published by the VHL Family Alliance, discusses the genetics of VHL in greater detail, and explains how you can compile family history information, which can be an important tool for your medical team. Family history information is important to understand your own condition, and to assist researchers in learning more about VHL.

Early Detection

Because VHL varies so widely, there is no consistent set of symptoms in each person. Each possible feature of the disease is detected in a different way.

If you have a family history of VHL, it is important to inform your doctor, or your child's pediatrician, and begin *screening* early, before any symptoms occur. Most VHL *lesions* are much easier to treat when they are small. Confer with your doctor about the best time to begin screening and the right schedule for return visits. We recommend informing the pediatrician of the family's history of VHL and beginning eye examinations for children at risk by age 1–3 years. You and your doctor may refer to Section 5, *Suggested Screening Guidelines*.

Nearly all of us at one time or another have wondered if it is better not to know — perhaps if we just don't go through the testing, we'll be okay. For a while, that may seem to be true. But a number of possible complications of VHL are sneaky — you may not even have symptoms until the problem has developed to a critical level. It is a little like not taking care of your house or car. You may get away with it for awhile, and then it all catches up with you and it costs you a great deal all at once. *There is clear, documented evidence that you will stay healthier longer if you use medical diagnostic techniques wisely and are watchful.*

> "I explain what's going on, how it works and what we're trying to fix, what could happen if it isn't fixed. I'm educating my patient in a way, but I'm also dispelling uncertainty. Uncertainty is the worst illness. The fear of the unknown can really be disabling."
> — Dr. Thomas Delbanco, Beth Israel Hospital, Boston, Massachusetts, as quoted in Bill Moyers, Healing and the Mind, *Doubleday Books, New York, 1993, p. 18.*

Detection of affected individuals by DNA analysis of a blood sample is now possible for nearly all VHL families. The accuracy of the testing, and its usefulness in most families, is increasing rapidly. DNA testing can be used to determine which members of the family need to be followed closely. It can also determine which members may be reassured that they do not carry the altered VHL gene. If family members do not have the altered VHL gene, they will not need further testing. They also cannot pass the altered gene to their children.

If you are a known VHL gene carrier, or if genetic testing does not yet work for your family, you will need to continue regular medical screening. One normal screening examination does not necessarily mean there is no VHL present, since the first evidence of VHL may occur later in life. Occasionally a person may be so mildly affected that VHL may seem to skip a generation. VHL has been diagnosed for the first time in people as old as 80, often because their children or grandchildren developed VHL tumors.

Even if there is no family history of VHL, when any one of the features of VHL is found a diagnosis of VHL should be considered and a full diagnostic evaluation of other areas of the body should be carried out. It is quite possible for someone to be the first in the family to have VHL. In some studies twenty percent of the patients were the first in their family to have VHL.

Depending on the outcome of your screening, your doctor will tell you what particular signs need to be followed closely. In general, vision problems, vomiting, headaches, balance problems, progressive weakness in arms or legs, or persistent pain lasting more than 1–2 days and that stays in one place, should be checked by your doctor.

Once VHL has been diagnosed in any one part of the body, it is important to undergo screening for possible evidences of the disease in other parts of the body, and to return for additional screening on the schedule recommended by your medical team.

> "My family has become convinced that one should never go alone to a doctor's appointment. If the news is difficult to hear, the brain shuts off at a certain point and just won't accept any more information. It helps if there are two people there, preferably with the unaffected person taking notes. If you have to go alone, take a tape recorder. You'll be amazed when you listen to the tape the next day."
> — *Darlene Y., Massachusetts*

General Recommendations for Screening

Your medical team will work with you to develop the right screening and monitoring program for you and your family.

Screening is testing before symptoms appear, to make sure that any issues are found early. See Section 5, *Suggested Screening Guidelines*.

Monitoring is checking up on known issues, to make sure that they are treated at the best time to insure long-term health. You and your medical team will work out the right interval for checkups, depending on your particular situation.

It is important to begin screening children who are at risk as early as possible. Using DNA testing, it is possible to identify which children need screening, and which children do not carry the VHL mutation and will not need to be screened.

The VHL Family Alliance and its medical advisors recommend that you begin screening children as early as age 1. **Make sure that the pediatrician knows that the child is at risk for VHL.** Eye examinations at this young age are particularly recommended.

Screening can be done using techniques that are not painful and do not involve radiation or contrast dyes: a thorough medical eye examination by a retinal specialist, and a complete physical examination including blood pressure and neurological examination, and hearing testing by an audiologist. Imaging of the brain, ultrasound of the abdomen, and often a 24-hour urine collection usually begin about age 10-12, or sooner if symptoms or signs occur. (See Figure 3.)

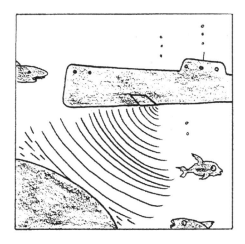

Figure 3: Ultrasound scanning. An Ultrasound scan works like the sonar used by submarines. Sound waves are sent out. A computer analyzes the reflection of the sound and calculates the depth and density of the tissue that reflects the sound. *Illustration by Vincent Giovannucci, O.D., Auburn, Massachusetts.*

Included in this booklet is a *Reminder Calendar* for you to record your own doctors' recommendations for screening or monitoring, the intervals recommended for repeat testing, and the date of your next appointments.

A *Suggested Screening Protocol,* or routine for checkups and treatment, is included in Section 5.

References:

Maher ER, Neumann HP, Richard S., von Hippel-Lindau disease: a clinical and scientific review. *Eur J Hum Genet*. 2011 Jun;19(6):617-23. Epub 2011 Mar 9. PMID: 21386872

Richard S, Lindau J, Graff J, Resche F. Von Hippel-Lindau disease. *Lancet*. 2004, 363:1231-4. PMID: 15081659

Lonser RR, Glenn GM, Chew EY, Libutti SK, Linehan WM, Oldfield EH, von Hippel-Lindau disease. *Lancet*. 2003 Jun 14;361(9374):2059-67. PMID: 12814730

> "In British parlance, patients are referred to as "sufferers."
> We'd like to change the British language.
> We are not sufferers, we are survivors.
> We are not victims, we are veterans.
> Just as the professionals have experience and expertise that we need and respect, we too have experience which is deserving of respect.
> Together with the physicians and researchers, we will succeed in our quest to improve diagnosis, treatment, and quality of life for people with von Hippel-Lindau. We are working to find a cure, but a cure will likely take decades. Meanwhile we are working through early diagnosis and improving treatment to manage this condition, and will do all we can to support one another through the experience."
> — *Joyce Graff, Co-Founder of the VHL Family Alliance, 1994*

Section 2:
Possible Manifestations

VHL in the Retina

When capillaries form angiomas, technically called hemangioblastomas, in the retina, they start out extremely small and difficult to see. The capillaries themselves are less than the diameter of a red blood corpuscle, one of the cells that make up the blood.

When angiomas begin, they often grow around the equator or periphery of the retina, far away from the area of central vision. Unlike the equator drawn around the globe of the world, the equator of the eye is vertical. As you stand, draw a circle around your eye from eyebrow to nose and around. The circle you just drew is the equator. To see this area, your *ophthalmologist* or *optometrist* must dilate your eye, use high-powered magnifying lenses, and look from side angles. It is more than the usual eye examination. (see Figure 4.) If there is VHL in your family, be sure to tell your ophthalmologist or optometrist so that he or she will be sure to do this thorough examination and find any small angiomas so that they can be treated in the early stages. A referral to a retinal specialist will be required for treatment of these tumors.

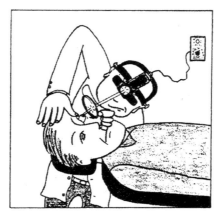

Figure 4: Ophthalmologist exploring the equator of the eye with indirect ophthalmoscope. *Illustration by Vincent Giovannuci, O.D.*

Not all ophthalmologists and optometrists are familiar with this uncommon disorder. You should look for an eye care professional who is familiar with VHL and qualified to perform a thorough dilated examination of the fundus and periphery with an indirect ophthalmoscope.

The objective of treatment is to keep the angioma so small that it does not affect your vision. Treatments generally include *laser treatment* (light surgery) or *cryotherapy* (freezing). Leaflets on these treatments are produced by the American Academy of Ophthalmology and other professional associations, and are usually available from your ophthalmologist. Both treatments are trying to keep the angioma from growing.

Sixty percent (60%) of people with VHL have retinal lesions. People as young as 3, and sometimes even younger, can be affected, making screening children very important. Children who have a positive DNA diagnosis of VHL should be screened for eye lesions beginning at age 1.

New angiomas can occur throughout life so that regular eye exams in affected individuals are important. Generally smaller lesions can be treated more successfully and with fewer complications than larger ones. Leakage or bleeding from larger angiomas can lead to serious vision damage or retinal detachment, so early treatment and careful management are very important.

Lesions on or near the optic nerve are very difficult to treat successfully and should not be approached with laser. Fortunately, they tend to grow slowly. Contact the VHL Family Alliance for the latest recommendations.

References:

American Academy of Ophthalmology, online brochures: "Laser Surgery in Ophthalmology," and "Cryotherapy," AAO, P.O. Box 7424, San Francisco, CA 94120-7424. 1 415 561-8500. http://www.aao.org

Chew, Emily, et al., von Hippel-Lindau disease: clinical considerations and the use of fluorescein-potentiated argon laser therapy for treatment of retinal angiomas. *Seminars in Ophthalmology.* 1992 Sep 7(3):182-91

The National Eye Institute (nei.nih.gov) and the National Library of Medicine (nlm.nih,gov) are both excellent resources for new terms and treatments

Dollfus H, Massin P, Taupin P, Nemeth C, Amara S, Giraud S, Beroud C, Dureau P, Gaudric A, Landais P, Richard S, Ocular manifestations in von Hippel-Lindau disease: a clinical and molecular study. *Invest. Ophthalmol. Vis Sci.* 2002, 43: 3067-74. PMID: 12202531

Gaudric A, Krisvosic V, Duguid G, Massin P, Giraud S, Richard S, Vitreoretinal surgery for severe retinal capillary hemanbioglastomas in von Hippel-Lindau disease. *Ophthamology.* 2011, 118: 142-9. PMID: 20801520

Wong WT, Chew EY. Ocular von Hippel-Lindau disease: clinical update and emerging treatments. *Curr Opin Ophthalmol.* 2008 May;19(3):213-7. Review. PMID: 18408496

VHL in the Brain and Spinal Cord

Angiomas in the brain and spinal cord are also called *hemangioblastomas*. A cyst inside the spinal cord is called a *syrinx*. When hemangioblastomas occur, they are generally not treated until symptoms begin to develop or unless they are growing rapidly. With regular visits to a *neurologist* on the schedule recommended by your medical team, early signs may be found which may then require further testing usually with MRI. Early signs and symptoms may include back pain, headaches, numbness, dizziness, and weakness or pain in the arms and legs. VHL brain tumors most commonly occur in the cerebellum.

Think of it as having a kind of wart on the inside. It's not a problem to have a wart unless it gets in your way. In these delicate areas, where there is little extra space, the problem is not so much having this wart, but rather the pressure it exerts on the brain tissue or the nerves in the spine. It is this pressure, or blockage of the normal flow of spinal fluid, which causes the symptoms. At the same time, some level of risk is associated with surgery to remove lesions of the brain or spinal cord, so the benefits and risks should be considered carefully. Surgery is usually advised after there are symptoms, but before the symptoms become severe.

Some new treatments are being tested. Occasionally, some minimally *invasive* treatment may be suggested at an early stage to stunt the growth of the tumor and prevent a cyst from forming. The objective, as in the eye, is to keep the *lesion* so small that it does not become a problem. Stereotactic radiosurgery, sometimes called by the name of the machine such as gamma knife or cyberknife, is a kind of treatment which does not require opening you up. Doctors focus beams of radiation from as many as 201 angles so that a high dose, or "zap" is delivered to a very tiny specific internal area where the beams meet. Some medical centers use stereotactic radiosurgery as a way of containing the growth of VHL brain tumors. It is sometimes helpful as a preventive, but not as a cure for an already symptomatic or advanced tumor. You may wish to discuss this option with your medical team. It will not be appropriate in every case. The approach to any brain or spinal hemangioblastoma needs to be discussed carefully with a *neurosurgeon* informed about VHL. (See next section, *Considering Stereotactic Radiosurgery.*)

Neither approach is always the right one. It depends on the particular tumor, its position and size, and the associated risks of each approach. It is important that you thoroughly understand the options, and that you work with your medical team to arrive at the right choice. Don't be shy to ask for second opinions. VHL or not, hemangioblastomas are rare tumors, and few surgeons have a great deal of experience with them. It is helpful both to you and to your neurosurgeon to have multiple opinions on the best approach to your problem.

References:

American Brain Tumor Association, "Dictionary for Brain Tumor Patients" and "A Primer of Brain Tumors," ABTA, 2720 River Road, Suite 146, Des Plaines, IL 60018. (800) 886-2282 or 1 708 827-9910; Fax: 1 708 827-9918. http://hope.abta.org info@abta.org

Ammerman JM, Lonser RR, Dambrosia J, Butman JA, Oldfield EH. Long-term natural history of hemangioblastomas in patients with von Hippel-Lindau disease: implications for treatment. *J Neurosurg.* 2006 Aug;105(2):248-55. PMID: 17219830

Peyre M., David P, Van Effenterre R, François P, Thus M., Emery E, Redondo A, Decq, P, Aghakhani N, Parker F, Tadié M., Lacroix C, Giraud S, Richard S. Natural history of supratentorial hemangioblastomas in von Hippel-Lindau disease. *Neurosurgery.* 2010, 67: 577-87. PMID: 20647972

Lonser, Russell R, et al., Surgical Management of CNS tumors in VHL. Series of articles concerning the specific sites of VHL tumors of the CNS. *J Neurosurgery.* 2003-2008. PMIDs: 12546358 (spinal), 12546357 (brain stem), 12859062 (nerve root), 18240914 (cerebellar)

Wind JJ, Lonser RR. Management of von Hippel-Lindau disease-associated CNS lesions. *Expert Rev Neurother.* 2011 Oct;11(10):1433-41. PMID: 21955200

Considering Stereotactic Radiosurgery

Stereotactic radiosurgery (SRS) is a non-invasive surgical technique similar to laser surgery, but using beams of radiation instead of light. Machines like the Gamma Knife, Cyberknife, Novalis, Proton Beam therapy, Stereotactic Linear Accelerator and other such machines are used to perform SRS. The marketing messages around the newest machines make it sound like magic, and it does work well for many kinds of tumors, but not for hemangioblastomas. For these vascular tumors, it can be at least as dangerous as open surgery. It is very important to approach SRS as you would any other surgical procedure — with healthy respect, caution, even skepticism. It is better to have the difficult conversation before, rather than after, the treatment. After 20 years of experience with SRS and hemangioblastoma, the VHL Family Alliance international team of medical advisors recommends:

- SRS not be used for hemangioblastomas of the brain unless the tumor has been deemed *unresectable* by a surgeon with experience in VHL, or unless the patient is in very poor health and could not sustain open surgery
- SRS not be used at all if the tumor is larger than 3 cubic centimeters (about 1.7 cm measured diagonally) or where a cyst is present, or when the patient is experiencing symptoms
- SRS not be used at all in the spinal cord or tissues other than brain, as this use is still experimental and there is insufficient data on effectiveness or possible complications

The best candidate tumor for SRS is a brain tumor less than 1.7 cm in size which does not have an associated cyst, and is not causing symptoms. It takes as long as two years to see the benefits of SRS treatment, and meanwhile the total mass of the tumor will increase before it begins to shrink. Patients who have symptoms or cysts usually need to have standard surgical resection.

Because SRS works best with small tumors, some of the tumors chosen for treatment might in fact never have grown. Most doctors prefer to wait until the tumor shows some signs of enlarging but without development of a cyst, before considering treatment with SRS.

The following list of questions has been assembled to help you have a discussion with your doctors about the wisdom of using SRS in your own situation. We don't want to alarm you, but we do want to make sure you and your doctor together examine all the possibilities prior to the treatment.

(1) Get both opinions. We strongly urge you to consult with a physician who is good at BOTH conventional micro-neurosurgery AND stereotactic radiosurgery. It is NOT enough to speak only with a radiation oncologist, interventional radiologist, or someone who practices only SRS. If you cannot find someone who practices both, be sure to talk with someone who is expert in the other method and get that perspective. In many cases, it is safer to approach a tumor with conventional surgery. You get it out, once and

for all, the tissue can be examined under a microscope, and the recovery period is better defined. Of course conventional surgery has its own set of risks and drawbacks, so you need a team of medical professionals who can help you evaluate fairly the pros and cons of both procedures and decide which is better for you in this particular situation at this particular time.

(2) How big is the tumor? Recommendations are NOT to treat a hemangioblastoma larger than 1.7 centimeters. Size is not the only issue, but it is a very important issue. Dr. Haring Nauta of the VHL Family Alliance Medical Advisory Board describes it like this: it's a matter of how finely you can focus the beams of radiation. It's rather like trying to burn a hole with a magnifying glass and sunlight. To make a small hole, you can focus the beam to a small point and use less radiation. To make a bigger hole, you have to cover a larger field, the beam is more weakly concentrated, and you have to use a lot more radiation to do the job. The tumor absorbs more energy and will swell more after the treatment.

(3) Is there a cyst or other source of mass effect? "Mass effect" is the effect of having some additional mass in your skull. This could be from a cyst, swelling, or from the tumor itself. If there is already extra pressure inside your skull, SRS is probably not a good idea, since the additional swelling caused by the procedure would compound the mass effect and make the symptoms worse.

(4) Where is it? Once treated, there will be swelling (*edema*) of the tumor and surrounding tissues. What this means to you is that the treated tumor will get bigger before it gets smaller, and depending how much room there is for it to expand, your symptoms may get worse before they get better. Where is the tumor located? When it swells, what symptoms may occur? How will the doctor propose to control the swelling? How can you work in partnership with the medical team to minimize the swelling and get through the swelling period? Note that this period of swelling is not measurable in days but in months. Ask your doctor how long you should expect this swelling period to last.

(5) What are the dangers to surrounding tissues? There is usually some margin of healthy tissue that will be irradiated with a therapeutic dosage. What tissue is within

that margin? What would such damage do? If the tumor is in a position where there is fluid beside it, then there is some "margin for error," but if it is in a critical spot, then its effect on the nearby healthy tissue can be significant.

(6) How many tumors do they propose to treat? What is the sum of the radiation to which you would be subjected? If more than one tumor is to be treated, is it wise to treat them all at this same time? Will the combined swelling of the various tumors cause a dangerous situation? Is it better to treat them one at a time? Pacing the treatment can be critical to managing the post-treatment swelling.

(7) What medication(s) would the doctor propose to use to manage the post-treatment period? Have you taken this medication before? Can they test you for sensitivity to the medication before the treatment, to make sure that you are not likely to have an adverse reaction? Some of the worst complications we have seen from stereotactic radiation involve sensitivities to the medication.

(8) What experience does this team have with treating hemangioblastoma, as opposed to solid tumors? Hemangioblastomas react differently to radiation treatment. It is important to get someone with experience in treating hemangioblastoma to participate in reviewing the treatment plan prior to the beginning of treatment. If you cannot find someone in your area, the VHL Family Alliance can suggest some sources of second opinions. This should be welcomed by your team, as it is for their protection as much as for your own.

References:

Asthagiri AR, Mehta GU, Zach L, Li X, Butman JA, Camphausen KA, Lonser RR. Prospective evaluation of radiosurgery for hemangioblastomas in von Hippel-Lindau disease. *Neuro Oncol.* 2010 Jan;12(1):80-6. Epub 2009 Dec 23. PMID: 20150370

Simone CB 2nd, Lonser RR, Ondos J, Oldfield EH, Camphausen K, Simone NL. Infratentorial craniospinal irradiation for von Hippel-Lindau: a retrospective study supporting a new treatment for patients with CNS hemangioblastomas. *Neuro Oncol.* 2011 Sep;13(9):1030-6. PMID: 21798886

Hearing Changes and VHL

The screening protocol includes a recommendation that you go regularly for an *audiometric* hearing examination. You should have a "baseline" study to document the state of your hearing, and periodically verify that it has not changed.

If you sense changes in your hearing or other indications of inner ear problems, you should follow up with a *neurotologist*. MRI of the Internal Auditory Canal should be used to check for an Endolymphatic Sac Tumor (ELST), which may occur in about 15% of people with VHL. The combined MRI recommended in the screening protocol is designed to monitor this area as well. (See Section 5, Suggested Screening Guidelines.)

An ELST forms in the endolymphatic sac, or in the temporal bone, behind the ear. The endolymphatic duct runs from the inner ear to the back surface of the petrous bone and ends beneath the dura at the boundary of the brain as a flattened expansion, the endolymphatic sac. (See Figure 5). This tiny structure is filled with fluid (called endolymph) and has a delicate system of pressure regulation that is responsible for one's sense of balance and equilibrium. Menière's disease is another condition that is caused by a disturbance in this area and causes similar symptoms (tinnitus, vertigo, hearing loss). ELSTs are often misdiagnosed as Menière's disease.

People report hearing changes which range from subtle changes in the "texture" of the hearing to profound hearing loss. Other symptoms may include hearing loss, tinnitus (ringing in the ears), dizziness, a fullness in the ears, or a weakness or slackness in the nerve that runs through the cheek of your face. Hearing loss may occur gradually over a period of 3–6 months or longer, or in some cases it may occur suddenly.

Once hearing is lost it is very difficult to regain. Here again, it is very important to watch for early symptoms and

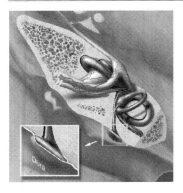

Figure 5. The inner ear, showing the endolymphatic sac (ELS).

The endolymphatic duct runs from the inner ear to the back surface of the petrous bone and ends beneath the dura at the boundary of the brain as a flattened expansion, the endolymphatic sac.

In the inset, you can see that the ELS is right up against the dura, the fibrous membrane that covers the brain. The bony structure is the petrous bone.

Fluid accumulation (called hydrops) may explain the Menière's-like symptoms (hearing loss, tinnitus, and vertigo) in patients with ELST. Hydrops may result from blockage of the reabsorption of endolymph in the endolymphatic sac, inflammation in response to hemorrhage, or excessive production of fluid by the tumor. Fluid production is typical also of other VHL tumors. *Illustration courtesy of Dr. Lonser, U.S. NIH. As published in* The VHL Family Forum, *12:2, September 2004.*

---

address the problem carefully in order to preserve hearing. If there is a loss of hearing, swift action will be needed if there is to be any hope of restoring it. If your local team is not familiar with ELST, please check with the nearest VHL Clinical Care Center, or with the VHL Family Alliance office, to get access to medical recommendations for action.

Once an ELST is visible on an MRI, surgery should be considered to prevent hearing loss, since swift action following hearing loss may not be possible. Careful surgical removal of the ELST will stop further damage and can usually be done without damaging hearing or balance. This delicate microsurgery usually requires teamwork between a neurosurgeon and a neurotologist in a practice that does a lot of inner ear surgery. Call the VHL Family Alliance for assistance in locating a surgeon familiar with this problem.

There are occasionally situations where the hearing may be affected even though no tumor or hemorrhage is visible on MRI. Tumors as small as 2 mm have been seen to affect hearing. Contact the VHL Family Alliance to get contact information for the team studying these very small tumors and developing recommendations for treatment.

There is one case reported where chronic ear infections were the first sign of an ELST in a 6-year-old. For this reason, if a child known to have VHL has ear infections, it would be advisable to do an MRI of the internal auditory canal before installing tubes in the ears, to potentially avoid ELST-associated hearing loss.

References:

Butman JA, et al., "Neurologic manifestations of von Hippel-Lindau disease, " *JAMA*. 2008 Sep 17;300(11):1334-42. PMID: 18799446

Choo, Daniel I, et al., "Endolymphatic Sac Tumors in von Hippel-Lindau Disease," *J Neurosurg*. 2004; 100:480-487. PMID: 15035284

Lonser, Russell R, et al., "Tumors of the Endolymphatic Sac in von Hippel-Lindau Disease," *N.E. J Med*. 2004; 350:2481-2486. PMID: 15190140

Megerian CA, Semaan MT. Evaluation and management of endolymphatic sac and duct tumors. *Otolaryngol Clin North Am*. 2007 Jun;40(3):463-78, viii. Review. PMID: 17544692

Kim M, Choi JY, et al., Hemorrhage in the endolymphatic sac: a cause of hearing fluctuation in enlarged vestibular aqueduct. *Int J Pediatr Otorhinolaryngol*. 2011 Dec;75(12):1538-44. PMID: 21963424

Kim HJ, Butman JA, Brewer C, Zalewski C, Vortmeyer AO, Glenn G, Oldfield EH, Lonser RR. Tumors of the endolymphatic sac in patients with von Hippel-Lindau disease: implications for their natural history, diagnosis, and treatment. *J Neurosurg*. 2005 Mar;102(3):503-12. PMID: 15796386

Poulsen ML, Gimsing S, Kosteljanetz M, Møller HU, Brandt CA, Thomsen C, Bisgaard ML. von Hippel-Lindau disease: Surveillance strategy for endolymphatic sac tumors. *Genet Med*. 2011 Dec;13(12):1032-41. PMID: 21912262

VHL and Your Reproductive Health

People with VHL should follow the cancer-preventive precautions and self-examinations recommended for everyone. Just because you have VHL does not exempt you from other conditions that occur in the general population. Follow the normal guidelines for breast and testicular self-examinations and take good care of your reproductive health. The VHL Family Alliance medical advisors also recommend that you consider vaccination against Human Papilloma Virus (HPV) as part of the usual preventive medical practice. While it is not directly involved in VHL, it is responsible for the promotion of several lethal cancers including cervical, vulvar, vaginal, penile, anal, and 30% of head and neck cancers. People should be vaccinated before they are sexually active, usually beginning about age 11-12.

There is one notable occurrence in men that is associated with VHL: epididymal cystadenomas may occur in as many as 50% of men with VHL. Similarly, women with VHL may have cystadenomas of the *broad ligament* near the *fallopian tube*, the *embryological* counterpart to the *epididymis*. Both are almost always harmless, although they may sometimes cause pain.

For Men

The epididymis is a small coiled conduit that lies above and behind the testicle, in the scrotum, on the path to the vas deferens, the tube that carries the sperm from the testicle to the prostate gland. The epididymis is as long as the testicle, lying in a flattened C shape against one side of the testicle. It's a complex tubular system that gathers the sperm and stores them until needed. It's a little like the coil on the back of an air conditioner, where the condensation takes place. (see Figure 6.) After having been stored in the epididymis, sperm then move through the vas deferens to the prostate, where they are mixed with seminal fluid from the seminal vesicles and move through the prostate into the urethra during ejaculation.

A small number of cysts are found in the epididymis of about one-fourth of men in the general population. By themselves, cysts are not an occasion for concern and are not even particularly noteworthy. However, one specific type of cyst is significant in VHL. A cystadenoma is a benign tumor with one or more cysts inside it, having more *density* than a simple cyst. *Papillary* cystadenomas of the epididymis are a rare occurrence in the general population. In VHL, these cysts can occur on one or both testes. When they occur on both sides, they almost always mean a definite diagnosis of VHL. They range in size from 1 to 5 centimeters (0.3 to 1.7 inches). The man may feel a "pebble" in the scrotum, but they are usually not painful and do not continue to enlarge.

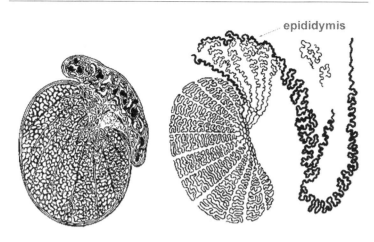

Figure 6: Epididymis. On the left, a cross-section through the testis and epididymis. On the right, the system of tubules of the testis and epididymis (see pointer). *Illustration by Gerhard Spitzer, after Rauber-Kopsch, from Kahle et al., Color Atlas, 2:261.*

Papllary cystadenomas of the epididymis may arise during the teenage years or later in life. It is not unusual for them to occur for the first time in men in their forties. The cysts can be removed if they are annoying. Removal is much the same operation as a vasectomy and may result in the disabling of the delivery of sperm from the operated side.

These cysts do not interfere with sexual function. In most cases the only "problem" associated with cystadenomas is the minor annoyance of knowing it is there. Occasionally, depending on their position, cystadenomas may block the delivery of sperm and cause infertility. If a cystadenoma is painful, you should definitely check with a doctor, since on rare occasions they can become inflamed and even rupture.

In some cases, they may cause atrophy of the vas deferens, which will also cause infertility. Men who wish to keep their childbearing options open may want to bank some sperm in their teens or twenties for possible later use.

The best way to keep track of epididymal cysts is to do a Testicular Self-Exam (TSE) monthly, as recommended for all men in the general population. VHL does not increase one's risk of testicular cancer. A TSE helps you become familiar with the size and shape of any epididymal cystadenomas, and make sure there are no unusual bumps or lumps in the testicles.

- Check yourself right after a hot shower. The skin of the scrotum is then relaxed and soft.
- Become familiar with the normal size, shape, and weight of your testicles.
- Using both hands, gently roll each testicle between your fingers.
- Identify the epididymis. This is a rope-like structure on the top and back of each testicle. This structure is NOT an abnormal lump, but epididymal cystadenomas may occur in this structure. Note their size and shape, and keep a record for comparison in the future.
- Be on the alert for a tiny lump under the skin, in front or along the sides of either testicle. A lump may remind you of a piece of uncooked rice or a small cooked pea.
- Report any swelling to your health care provider.

If you have lumps or swellings, it does not necessarily mean that you have testicular cancer, but you must be checked by your healthcare provider.

References:

Odrzywolski KJ, Mukhopadhyay S., "Papillary cystadenoma of the epididymis," *Arch Pathol Lab Med.* 2010 Apr;134(4):630-3. PMID: 20367315

Aydin H, Young RH, Ronnett BM, Epstein JI, "Clear cell papillary cystadenoma of the epididymis and mesosalpinx: immunohistochemical differentiation from metastatic clear cell renal cell carcinoma," *Am J Surg Pathol.* 2005 Apr;29(4):520-3. PMID: 15767808T

Ernesto Fugueroa, M.D., How to Perform a Testicular Self-Examination, kidshealth.org, Alfred I. DuPont Hospital, Wilmington, DE, and Jefferson Medical Center, Philadelphia

For Women

A corresponding tumor occurs in women, called an Adnexal Papillary Cystadenoma of Probable Mesonephric Origin (APMO). A cystadenoma is a benign tumor with one or more cysts inside it, having more *density* than a simple cyst. *Papillary* cystadenoma of the broad ligament are a rare occurrence in the general population.

The broad ligament is a folded sheet of tissue that drapes over the uterus, fallopian tubes and the ovaries. (See Figure 7.) Cells in this area are from the same origin in the development of the embryo as the epididymis in males.

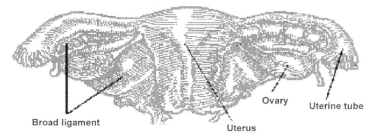

Figure 7: Broad ligament. The broad ligament is a large area of tissue that lies on top of the reproductive organs in women. The broad ligament looks like drapery material, lying in folds and creases on top of both ovaries and uterine tubes, connecting these structures to the uterus. Some of the cystadenomas that occur in VHL will be found attached to adnexal (adjoining) tissue that is not part of the broad ligament, sometimes below it. These are called adnexal papillary cystadenoma of probable mesonephric duct origin (APMO). *Illustration by Frank James.*

Cysts in this area are very common in the general population. However if an "unusual" cyst or tumor is seen in the area of the broad ligament or fallopian tubes, a cystadenoma associated with VHL should be considered. Ask your doctor to do a careful differential diagnosis to prevent over-treatment of benign tumors, as they are sometimes confused with ovarian cancer.

Please report tumors of the broad ligament or fallopian tube to the VHL Family Alliance research database to help expand our knowledge about this condition. Until more is known about this VHL associated tumor, the reviewing call these tumors by another name such [as tu]mors of low *malignant* potential."

[There is] still no definitive recommendations on birth [control. S]ince there are progesterone receptors on VHL [tumors, the Fr]ench VHL Study Group recommends choosing a birth control pill with lower levels of progesterone.

References:

James, G. P., Hastening the Road to Diagnosis: the Role of the Broad Ligament Cystadenoma in Early Detection of VHL. *VHL Family Forum*. 1998, www.vhl.org/newsletter/vhl1998/98ccapmo.php or search for "James and APMO"

Janovski NA, Bozzetti LP, "Serous Papillary Cystadenoma arising in Paramesonephric rest of the mesosalpinx," *Obstet Gynecol*. 1963 Nov;22:684-7. PMID: 14082297

Zanotelli DB, Bruder E, Wight E, Troeger C., "Bilateral papillary cystadenoma of the mesosalpinx: a rare manifestation of von Hippel-Lindau disease," *Arch Gynecol Obstet*. 2010 Sep;282(3):343-6. Epub 2010 Feb 16. PMID: 20157715

Pregnancy and VHL

Women with VHL should take special precautions when considering pregnancy. Research by the French VHL Study Group seems to indicate that pregnancy may promote some additional tumor growth, especially in the eye, brain, and spinal cord. At the least, it does not halt tumor growth, and a woman's childbearing years are also a time when tumors are likely to grow. All the changes in your body during pregnancy can mask symptoms and signs of tumors, so it is important to know what is going on before those changes begin, and to monitor progress during the pregnancy, including an MRI without contrast in the fourth month of pregnancy.

- Your blood volume will double during pregnancy. If you have a hemangioblastoma in the brain, spinal cord or retina, this increased blood flow may expand the tumor at least for a period of time during the pregnancy. Some women have reported worsening of symptoms during the pregnancy, followed by a lessening of symptoms after delivery. In some cases the expansion took mild or non-existent symptoms and expanded them to a critical level.

- The weight of the fetus will add strain to your spinal column. Depending on what tumors are already present in the spinal cord, this additional stress may cause a worsening of symptoms.
- The additional fluids will put increased load on your kidneys. You need to make sure that your kidney function is normal so that your kidneys will serve you and your baby well.
- The stress of pregnancy and delivery can trigger an existing pheochromocytoma (pheo). (See next section, *Blood Pressure, Emotions, and VHL*.) Be very sure to get checked — and re-checked — for a pheo during the pregnancy, to avoid these complications.

If you are considering getting pregnant, or if you have already become pregnant, have a thorough check-up in order to identify any tumors you may already have. Discuss with your doctor what might happen if these tumors should grow during pregnancy. Since it is preferable not to use tests that involve radiation while you are pregnant for fear of harming the baby, it is best if you can do the testing in advance and know what your risk factors are. Hopefully the tumors will not grow, but if they do, here are some things you should discuss with your obstetrician and other medical specialists:

- What symptoms should you watch for?
- Would the consequences possibly have a serious impact on your own health?
- How could it affect the fetus?

In particular, get a thorough test for a *pheochromocytoma* ("pheo" (say FEE-oh) for short). It is critically important that you be tested for a pheo before planning a pregnancy, or as soon as you are pregnant, and especially before going through the birthing process. An active pheo can be life-threatening to you and your baby.

Discuss these risk factors fully with your partner as well before making the decision. This is a joint decision. You might be willing to risk it, but is your partner willing to put you at risk? Discussing it prior to pregnancy is much better than living with the anger or guilt that can arise from walking blindly into a risky situation.

If you are already pregnant, tell your obstetrician and connect him or her with other members of your medical team. Watch for symptoms and report any symptoms to the doctor. Vomiting and headaches will take more watching than for most pregnant women, since these can also be signs of brain and spinal tumors. Don't ignore them or discount them, particularly if they are excessive or persistent. A little morning sickness is normal; the amount of vomiting is variable within a pregnancy, and you should always check with your medical team on whether there is cause for concern. Don't panic; talk with your doctors.

It is recommended that you have an MRI — without contrast — during the fourth month of pregnancy, especially if you have known tumors of the brain or spinal cord, to check on any change in these lesions.

If you have eye, brain or spinal lesions, a C-section should be considered, to avoid pushing during labor which might aggravate these lesions.

Approximately 2–3 months after the baby is born, have another thorough check-up to evaluate any changes in your own health.

References:

El-Sayed, Yasser, Pregnancy and VHL. *VHL Family Forum.* 2001, www.vhl.org/newsletter/vhl2001/01eapreg.htm

Lenders J, "Endocrine disorders in pregnancy: Phaeochromocytoma and pregnancy: a deceptive connection," *Eur J Endocrinol.* 2011 Sep 2. PMID: 21890650

Abadie C, Coupier I, Bringuier-Branchereau S, Mercier G, Deveaux S, Richard S. The role of pregnancy on hemangioblastomas in von Hippel-Lindau disease: a retrospective French study. *9th International Symposium on VHL,* Rio de Janeiro (Brazil). 2010 Oct 21–24. Journal article in press

Pre-Implantation Genetic Diagnosis

With the advances in genetic testing, there is a new technology that couples may wish to consider in order to know if the embryo carries the VHL alteration. In-vitro fertilization (IVF), or fertilization of the egg and sperm, is performed in the laboratory. Two days after fertilization a single cell is teased out of the developing embryo. The single cell sample is sent to a genetics lab for analysis. Usually samples from at least 4–8 developing embryos are analyzed; the results specify which of the embryos are affected with the VHL alteration, and which are not. A small number of unaffected embryos can then be implanted into the woman's uterus and the pregnancy proceeds forward normally. Embryos not implanted can be frozen for future use.

It takes pre-planning to accomplish this, since the DNA testing must be accomplished is a very short time. Before the IVF process can be started, samples of DNA from both parents and sometimes also from other close relatives must be sent to the DNA testing lab, and a test prepared for analyzing the VHL status of the embryonic sample. Once the test is ready, the IVF process can be started. It is now possible to develop such a genetic test for most VHL mutation types, though not all.

If you would like to explore this option, you should make contact with a certified Fertility Clinic offering In-Vitro Fertilization with optional Pre-implantation Genetic Diagnosis (PGD). Men who have previously banked sperm can use IVF to have a child, with or without PGD.

IVF-PGD is not a trouble-free process. It may take several cycles before it succeeds. There are difficulties and disappointments along the path. Nonetheless, as of 2012, there are ten healthy babies known to have been born to VHL-affected couples through this technology.

Women with VHL who choose this path are asked to share their information and experiences so that more can be learned about any special concerns around the hormone injections required for this process. Please contact the VHL Family Alliance for referral to the international team leading this effort, to get their current request for data.

Some anonymous articles have been published in the VHL Family Forum describing some couples' experiences with various childbearing choices, including PGD. See "childbearing choices" at vhl.org.

Blood Pressure, Emotions, and VHL

VHL may be associated with a kind of tumor of the adrenal glands called a *pheochromocytoma*, ("*pheo*"). The adrenal glands are approximately 3 x 2 x 2 cm (1 inch long) perched on top of each of the kidneys. (See Figure 8.) These tumors occur more frequently in some families than in others. They are rarely malignant (3%) among people with VHL. Detected early, they are not difficult to deal with, but they are potentially lethal if not treated because of the damage they can cause to the heart and blood vessels and the potential for dangerously high blood pressure occurring during stresses such as surgery, accidents, or childbirth.

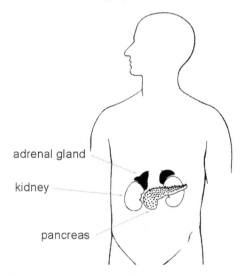

Figure 8. Kidney, pancreas, and adrenal glands. The figure shows the relative positions of these organs. *Illustration by Gerhard Spirzer, from Kahle et al., Color Atlas, 2:141.*

Pheos produce so-called "stress hormones" (noradrenaline and adrenaline) that your body uses to gain speed and strength in an emergency. The pheo secretes excessive amounts of these stress hormones into the bloodstream. The primary symptom is usually high blood pressure, especially spiking blood pressure, that puts strain on your heart and vascular system and can cause heart attack or stroke. In some patients, though, blood pressure may be normal. Patients may notice headache, irregular or rapid heartbeat, or what feels like a panic attack, fear, anxiety or sometimes rage. There may be heavy sweating for no good reason. Sometimes people have hot flashes (or cold flashes). There may be abdominal pain, or unexplained weight loss. It is recommended that all people with VHL be screened for pheos. New research indicates that adrenal tumors are as much as four times more common among people with VHL than previously thought. Even in families that have not previously had a pheo, it is still important to test for presence of these tumors. In one large progeny in France where there were no pheos for three generations, there are now pheos in two branches of that family. (Richard, 2011.)

Traditional blood or urine tests that measure only catecholamines are inadequate to find most pheos. Usually an initial biochemical test is done to measure blood or urine metanephrines, and if additional information is required, or if there are symptoms of pheo but the blood and urine tests are negative, anatomical imaging scans may be used. It is particularly important to be checked for a pheo prior to any surgery, pregnancy, or childbirth. If a pheo is present, complications may be avoided by blocking off the effects of stress hormones with drugs, beginning at least 7–14 days before the procedure.

The accuracy of the urine and blood tests for pheochromocytoma activity will be determined in large part by your own cooperation in preparing for the test. Even if no instructions are provided, you should avoid smoking, alcohol, and caffeine for at least four hours before the test. Be sure to tell your doctor and the technician if you are taking any anti-depressant or mood-altering medication. You might want to prepare a list of all the medications you are taking, discuss this list with the doctor before the test, and even send it along to the lab with the blood or urine sample, to assist in interpreting the results. Where other instructions are given, they may differ from center to center, sometimes due to different methods of analysis. Follow any instructions carefully to avoid a false reading. See *Preparing for Pheo Testing* in Section 5.

Pheos often cause symptoms that may lead you or your doctor to believe you are having a heart attack or stroke. That is because the chemicals produced by the pheo cause your cardiovascular system to go into overdrive. If beta blockers are prescribed, they often make the symptoms worse. This is further indication that you should be tested for a pheo.

Pheos often cause symptoms that may lead you or your doctor to believe you are having psychological symptoms. Medications are often recommended, or self-prescribed. It is important to note that all medications may interfere with the accurate analysis of tests for pheo. If at all possible, testing for pheo should be done BEFORE beginning any medication. If this is not possible, then it is critically important that you disclose ALL medications you are taking — prescription, herbal, over-the-counter, and even illegal — in order to get an accurate reading from the tests. Such medications can interfere with the results, depending on the method of measurement used by the laboratory. Please adhere to any recommendations about medication indicated to you by the laboratory or your physician. See *Preparation for Pheo Testing* in Section 5.

The preferred test for a pheo is a "plasma-free metanephrines" test. This involves measurement in a sample of blood of both metanephrine, the metabolite of adrenaline, and normetanephrine, the metabolite of noradrenaline. Slightly less accurate but more widely available is the 24-hour urine collection, analyzed for fractionated metanephrines, normetanephrine, and metanephrine.

In VHL, it is only necessary to consider elevations of normetanephrine. For plasma in an adult patient with VHL, anything over 112 pg/mL (0.61 nmol/L, the NIH upper reference limit) should evoke suspicion. Anything over 400 pg/mL (2.2 nmol/L) for a sample that is taken with the patient lying down and relaxed (no stress) and on no antidepressants is immediately highly suspicious (close to 100% likelihood) and imaging is warranted. Between those ranges the likelihood of a pheo increases with increased level and follow-up tests should be considered.

If these chemical tests indicate the presence of a pheo, but it cannot easily be located on MRI or CT, an MIBG or PET scan may be recommended. These scans help to *localize*, or locate, a pheo, even if it is outside the adrenal glands.

Pheos located outside the adrenal glands are sometimes called *paragangliomas*. They may occur anywhere on the sympathetic nervous system, meaning anywhere along a line drawn from your groin to your ear lobe, on either side of the body. Multiple tests may be needed to find them. According to research at the U.S. National Institutes of Health, different tests have different success rates in locating a pheochromocytoma or paraganglioma:

- ^{18}F-FDA PET finds 75–92%
- ^{18}F-FDOPA PET finds 67–93%
- ^{123}I-MIBG scan finds 67–86%
- ^{18}F-FDG PET finds 83–93% (adrenal: 67%)
- Octreoscan finds fewer than 50% of these tumors

The choice of one of these tests is often made depending on the availability of a particular technology at your center. However it is important to note that if the test chosen does not find the pheo, there is still some chance that the pheo is in fact there, but cannot be detected by that particular test. You may need to seek a second opinion from a VHL expert.

If surgery is required, the standard of care these days is partial *adrenalectomy*. Studies have shown that keeping even a small amount of the cortex of the adrenal gland will make it much easier for you to manage after surgery and usually avoid steroid replacement. Thus even if you still have another healthy gland, remember that there may be another pheo in the future that could put that second gland at risk, so your goal should be to keep a portion of each gland working for you.

In recent years the "key hole" operating technique (*laparoscopy*) is being used to treat pheos. Laparoscopic partial adrenalectomy is now possible in most cases. With this technique there is less risk of infection, and the recovery is much faster. You may wish to discuss the references below with your doctor.

Prior to surgery they will prescribe "blockers" (alpha blockers, sometimes followed by beta blockers) to calm the effects of the chemicals produced by the pheo, and allow the surgery to proceed calmly, without causing a pheo crisis. The blockers will make you tired, but they are critically important. They may be prescribed for two or more weeks before the planned surgery. See also Section 5.

References:

Asher, KP, et al., Robot-assisted laparoscopic partial adrenalectomy for pheochromocytoma: the National Cancer Institute technique, *Eur Urol.* 2011 Jul;60(1):118-24. Epub 2011 Apr 9. PMID: 21507561

Germain A, et al., Surgical management of adrenal tumors, *J Visc Surg.* 2011 Sep;148(4):e250-61. Epub 2011 Aug 5. PMID: 21820984

Kantorovich V, Eisenhofer G, Pacak K, Pheochromocytoma: an endocrine stress mimicking disorder, *Ann N Y Acad Sci.* 2008 Dec;1148:462-8. PMID: 19120142

Pacak K. G. Eisenhofer, and J. Timmers. Pheochromocytoma. In J.L. Jameson and L.S. DeGroot, (eds) *Textbook of Endocrinology.* 6th edition. Elsevier Science Inc., Philadelphia, 2010

Stéphane Richard, presentation at the 4th International Symposium on Pheochromocytoma, Paris 2011

Yousef HB, et al., Laparoscopic vs open adrenalectomy: experience at King Faisal Specialist Hospital and Research Centre, Riyadh, *Ann Saudi Med.* 2003 Jan-Mar; 23(1-2):36-8. PMID: 17146220

VHL in the Kidneys

The kidneys are organs about 12 cm (4 inches) long in the abdominal cavity, or about the size of your fist. (See Figure 8.) VHL in the kidney may cause cysts or tumors. It is common for any adult in the general population to have an occasional kidney cyst. VHL cysts are usually multiple, but the presence of one or more simple cysts is not a problem in itself. It is also possible for tumors to form in the kidney that are *renal cell carcinomas (RCC),* one kind of kidney *cancer,* formerly known as *hypernephroma.*

There are generally no specific physical signs to help find problems early. It is critically important to begin monitoring the kidneys long before any obvious physical symptoms or signs occur. The kidneys continue to function while these structural changes are occurring, without physical symptoms, and with normal urine tests.

Think of it as having a mole on your skin, except that you cannot see that it is growing. When it is very small there may be no cause for alarm. When the mole begins to grow or change in suspicious ways your doctor would recommend that it be removed.

Similarly, when a kidney tumor is quite large when discovered, or if it changes shape, or its size or rate of growth becomes suspicious, your medical team may recommend surgery. Not all kidney tumors require immediate surgery. Based on characteristics such as density, size, shape, and location, they will recommend either a time to repeat the imaging tests or surgical *resection* (removal of the tumor). Once they emerge, VHL kidney tumors are like Clear Cell Renal Cell Carcinoma (ccRCC) in the general population. The biggest difference is that in VHL we have the opportunity to find them earlier than most people who have *sporadic* kidney cancer. That gives us much better options for dealing with them early, keeping that kidney working for you, and avoiding the worst consequences of cancer. Knowing that someone with VHL is at risk for RCC, the tumors can be found at much earlier stages. If you wait for symptoms, the tumor will usually be at a much later and more dangerous stage when it is found.

Opinions differ on the right time to operate, but there is widespread agreement on this general approach. In VHL, a person with kidney involvement typically has a series of tumors on both kidneys over the course of several decades. Clearly one cannot remove every little tumor, since that would be too many surgeries for the person, and especially for this small organ, to endure. The goal is to maintain the patient's own kidney function throughout his or her lifetime, to minimize the number of surgeries and yet remove tumors before they *metastasize* and cause the cancer to grow in other organs. The tricky part is to choose the right moment to operate—not too early and not too late.

The objective is to track the progression of the cells from harmless to a later point, but before they become capable of spreading. If you think of a dandelion, it begins as a bud, becomes a rather pretty yellow flower, turns white, and one day the white seedlings are carried off on the wind to seed the lawn. If you pick the yellow flowers, the seeds are not mature and cannot spread. The cells have to mature to the point where they know how to seed themselves in the lawn. The trick to living with dandelions is to pick them while they are yellow.

There is a similar transition in cancer. Cancer researchers have identified a series of distinct stages that the cells go through before they are even capable of metastasizing.

It would be ideal if there were some easy blood or urine test—some *biomarker*—to check on the cell progression. There is no such test at this time, though there is a great deal of research effort to find one. Meanwhile, clinical research has shown that the size of a solid tumor is one relatively crude but fairly reliable sign of its progress.

Biopsies are usually not called for in this case, since with a diagnosis of VHL one is pretty certain what the structure will contain. There will be cancer cells even in very small tumors. The question is: what is their level of progression? This is not a question that can be answered accurately through a biopsy.

Cysts are generally not considered sufficient cause for an operation. There will be a small seedling of a tumor in the wall of the cyst, and it will be important to watch the size of that tumor, not of the cyst itself.

The consensus from the Freiburg (Germany) meeting (1994) was to recommend surgery only when the largest tumor is larger than 3 cm. This recommendation was verified by a multi-center study under Dr. Andrew Novick. (Steinbach, 1995.) All the VHL study teams worldwide now concur with this guideline. After nearly 20 years of experience using these guidelines, there are only three verified reports of metastasis from tumors smaller than 4 cm, all of which were at or greater than 3 cm.

In watching your kidneys, your medical team is working to evaluate whether you have cysts or solid tumors. You will need tests such as *magnetic resonance imaging* (MRI) or *computed tomography* (CT). The doctors will watch the tissue density, the position of the tumors, their size and rate of growth. MRI is preferred in most cases, as it does not use radiation.

It is important that you understand in as much detail as you can the medical findings that your medical team is concerned about, so that you can participate with them in determining the right timing and treatment. Don't be shy to get a second opinion. The distinction between a cyst and a tumor can be debatable depending on the clarity of the image and the experience of the *radiologist* who reviews the VHL tumors. Even among experts there can be differences of opinion. This is an area where the perspective of one or more physicians with significant experience in VHL can make a world of difference. Films or compact discs (CDs) can easily be sent to a consulting physician far away, even in another country. Contact the VHL Family Alliance for assistance in locating an expert who can assist you.

Decisions about when to operate and the extent of the procedure need to be made by the entire team, especially including the patient, with full disclosure of all information. All points of view, the location of the tumor, the patient's level of stamina and health, and even the possible desire of the patient to be free of the tumor, all play a role.

In cases where the last remaining kidney must be removed, VHL patients have been proven to be good candidates for kidney transplant. (See Goldfarb, 1997.) VHL tumors grow from abnormalities within the cells of the kidney itself. Since the new kidney has the donor's genetic structure and two healthy copies of the VHL gene, it is not at risk for VHL tumors. Immune suppression for transplantation has not been seen to increase the growth of other VHL tumors.

References:

Duffey, B. G., Choyke, P. L., Glenn, G., Grubb, R. L., Venzon, D., Linehan, W. M., and Walther, M. M. The Relationship Between Renal Tumor Size and Metastases in Patients with von Hippel-Lindau Disease. *J Urol.* 172: 63-65, 2004. PMID: 15201738

Goldfarb DA, et al., "Results of renal transplantation in patients with renal cell carcinoma and von Hippel-Lindau disease," *Transplantation,* 1997 Dec 27;64(12):1726-9. PMID: 9422410

Matin SF, et al., "Patterns of intervention for renal lesions in von Hippel-Lindau disease," *BJU Int.* 2008 Sep; 102(8):940-5. Epub 2008 May 15. PMID: 18485044

Joly D., Méjean A, Corréas JM, Timsit MO, Verkarre V, Deveaux S, Landais P, Grünfeld JP, Richard S. Progress in nephron-sparing therapy of renal cell carcinoma and von Hippel-Lindau disease. *J Urol.* 2011, 185:2056-60. PMID: 21496837

Shuch B, et al., "Repeat partial nephrectomy: surgical, functional, and oncological outcomes," *Curr Opin Urol.* 2011 Sep; 21(5):368-75. doi: 10.1097/MOU.0b013e32834964ea. PMID: 21788903

VHL in the Pancreas

The pancreas is an organ extending from left to right in the upper abdomen, in the back, lying directly behind and against the stomach and the small intestine. (See Figure 8.) It consists of two glandular parts: one produces secretions which are essential in digestion, which flows by way of the large pancreatic duct together with bile produced by the *liver* into the upper part of the digestive tract. The other part is formed by the islet cells, in which hormones such as insulin are formed. Insulin is the hormone that regulates the blood sugar level.

Pancreatic lesions are generally considered to be the least *symptomatic* among the lesions of von Hippel-Lindau disease. Families report a number of subtle symptoms, though, which may be caused by pancreatic cysts.

Three types of lesions may be found commonly in the pancreas:

- cysts
- *serous microcystic adenomas*, or "cystadenomas"
- islet cell tumors, or pancreatic neuroendocrine tumors (NET)

Pancreatic cysts may be found in a large number of people with VHL, with wide variation among families. About 75% of people with VHL will develop pancreatic cysts. Many cysts, even very large ones, may be present without causing symptoms, in which case no treatment is required. In some cases, enlarged cysts may press against the stomach and cause discomfort. Surgical drainage of a large cyst may provide relief.

About 12% of people with VHL may develop one of two kinds of tumors in the pancreas. *Serous microcystic adenomas,* benign tumors, are the most common. These generally need not be removed unless they are causing obstructions to the normal flow of fluids and enzymes that cannot be managed otherwise.

Depending on their size, type and location, VHL cysts and tumors of the pancreas can cause functional problems as well as structural problems. Your medical team may request additional tests to detect abnormal hormonal function. The job of the pancreas is to create hormones and enzymes that are important to the digestion of the food you eat, making the nutrients in the food available to your cells. Cysts and tumors may block one or more of the ducts that carry essential fluids from the pancreas to the digestive tract, causing diarrhea, constipation, fatty stools, other digestive complaints, and weight loss. Blockage of the delivery of insulin may cause digestive problems or diabetes. Fortunately, there are replacements that can be taken by pill or injection. Insulin or digestive enzymes may need to be prescribed to maintain health. Figuring how much of which enzyme you need at what times is not an easy thing to calculate. A gastroenterologist or naturopath familiar with pancreatic insufficiency and digestive imbalance can assist you in achieving the right balance to improve your quality of life.

If lesions obstruct the bile ducts, there may be jaundice, pain, inflammation or infection. Jaundice is when the skin and urine become yellow, and the stools become quite pale. Pain is your body's signal to you that there is something wrong that requires attention; seek medical help immediately, as *pancreatitis* is a serious condition requiring medical attention.

The most worrisome pancreatic issue is solid tumors, not cysts, arising within the islet cells of the pancreas, which may be pancreatic neuroendocrine tumors (*Pancreatic NET*). They can cause bile duct obstructions, and can even metastasize or spread to the liver or bone.

Some of the "hard tumors" turn out to be microcystic adenomas, honeycombed clusters of small cysts, that look solid on the scans but in fact are not a problem.

Careful evaluation of pancreatic NETs is important, as it would be best not to operate on the pancreas unless it is important to do so. Pancreatic NETs are not "functional" in VHL, meaning they do not emit hormones, so chemical tests will not help to determine their nature.

A 12-year study at the U.S. National Institutes of Health under Dr. Steven Lubutti (see Blansfield, 2007) identified three variables that are important in deciding whether intervention is required: size, behavior, and the nature of the DNA alteration.

Size has traditionally been our primary indicator, and it continues to be important. Any "hard tumor" (pancreatic NET) larger than 2 cm needs to be taken very seriously.

- *DNA:* They found a higher correlation of dangerous Pancreatic NETs among people who have an alteration in Exon 3 of the VHL gene. The VHL gene has three distinct parts, called Exons. Each family has a particular mutation, like a misspelling of one word in the book of instructions that make up the VHL protein. That family mutation is passed intact from parent to child, so each family member has the same alteration in their VHL gene. People with a mutation in Exon 3 seem to have a more aggressive type of pancreatic tumor.

- *Behavior:* They also looked for signs of aggressive behavior. To measure aggressiveness, they took a series of images and compared the size of the largest tumor in each of these scans, then calculated its rate of growth, or "doubling rate". If the tumor doubled in size in less than 500 days, it was deemed to be high risk. If it took longer than 500 days for the tumor to double, it was at a more moderate risk level.

- *Size:* In the past, recommendations for when to operate have been based entirely on size. But now, with the addition of these new measures, Libutti has divided tumors into three categories — low risk tumors can be watched every 2-3 years; medium risk tumors should be followed more closely, and high-risk tumors should be evaluated for surgery. (see Table 1.)

Table 1: Assessing the risk level of a pancreatic neuroendocrine tumor.
Source: "Clinical, genetic and radiographic analysis of 108 patients with von Hippel-Lindau disease (VHL) manifested by pancreatic neuroendocrine neoplasms (PNETs)." by Blansfield JA, Libutti SK, et al., *Surgery.* 2007 Dec;142(6):814-8; discussion 818.e1-2.

High risk - evaluate for surgery	Medium risk - follow until a second criterion is present	Low risk - follow every 2-3 years
Size >= 3 cm	Size 2-3 cm.	Size < 2 cm.
Mutation in exon 3	Mutation in exon 1 or 2	Mutation in exon 1 or 2
Doubling in <500 days		

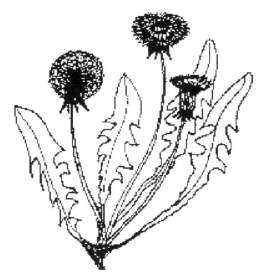

Figure 9: Dandelions demonstrate that cells need to mature to a certain point before they know how to send out seeds and plant more tumors in other places. We need not pull up every green one, but it is important to pick them while they are yellow. To manage VHL, you and your medical team will work out the right balance between avoiding metastatic cancer and maintaining healthy organs.

References:

Blansfield JA, , Choyke L, Morita SY, Choyke PL, Pingpank JF, Alexander HR, Seidel G, Shutack Y, Yuldasheva N, Eugeni M, Bartlett DL, Glenn GM, Middelton L, Linehan WM, and Libutti SK. Clinical, genetic and radiographic analysis of 108 patients with von Hippel-Lindau disease (VHL) manifested by pancreatic neuroendocrine neoplasms (PNETs). *Surgery.* 2007 Dec;142(6):814-8; discussion 818.e1-2. PMID: 18063061

Corcos O, Couvelard A, Giraud S, Vullierme MP, O'Toole D, Rebours V, Stievenart JL, Penfornis A, Niccoli-Sire P, Baudin E, Sauvanet A, Lévy P, Ruszniewski P, Richard S, Hammel P. Endocrine pancreatic tumors in von Hippel-Lindau disease: clinical, histological and genetic features. *Pancreas.* 2008. 37:85-93. PMID: 18580449

Hammel P, Vilgrain V, Terris B, Penfornis A, Sauvanet A, Corréas, JM, Chauveau D, Balian A, Beigelman C, O'Toole D, Mernardes P, Ruszniewski P, Richard S. Pancreatic involvement in von Hippel-Lindau disease: prevalence, course and impact in the management of patients. *Gastroengerology.* 2000, 119: 1087-1095. PMID: 11040195

Section 3:
Diagnosis, Treatment, and Research
Diagnosis and Treatment

Your medical team will advise you on the best diagnostic tests to use, and the best course of treatment for the VHL involvement shown by your screening. There are a number of very effective treatments, and more are being discovered.

In addition to physical examination by your doctor, evaluation of suspicious areas will probably involve some combination of magnetic resonance imaging (MRI), computed tomography (CT) scanning, ultrasound scanning, and angiography. The objective is to provide diagnostic pictures of both the blood vessels and soft tissues of your body. This may involve injecting contrast materials, or dyes, into your bloodstream to help the doctors see the blood vessels more clearly in the pictures. Various techniques are also used to determine the *density* of the tissues being examined, which helps the medical team determine whether it is normal tissue, cyst, or tumor.

Positron Emission Tomography (PET) scanning may be used to determine the activity level of certain kinds of tumors.

Treatments usually involve some kind of surgery to remove potentially malignant tumors before they become harmful to other tissues. Evaluation of a surgical alternative is always a matter of choosing the lesser of two evils. Surgery always has some level of risk, but keeping the angioma or tumor also has its risks. Advances are providing surgical alternatives that are less *invasive*, but newer is not necessarily better. You should discuss the relative risks with your medical team.

Even the list of risks that the anesthesiologist reads off before surgery can sound frightening. It is sometimes helpful to say to the doctor, "What odds would you give me of one of those things happening?" Finding out that they are reading a list of things, all of which add up to less than 4%, as opposed to a risk level of 50%, helps to put the risk into perspective. Each of us must examine the relative benefits and risks of a proposed surgery in consultation with our medical teams.

Genetic Research and VHL

DNA (deoxyribonucleic acid) is the biochemical basis of life and of heredity. All of an individual's characteristics are written in DNA in a kind of code. DNA is assembled into microscopic structures called *chromosomes*. In the human species there are 46 chromosomes, 23 from the mother and 23 from the father. There are 22 *autosomes*, numbered 1 to 22, of which each person has a pair (two copies of chromosome 1, two of chromosome 2, etc...) and one pair of the "sex" chromosomes, XX for females and XY for males. On each chromosome are the genes that contain the specific information necessary for the manufacture of proteins. Each gene has two copies, one inherited from the father, and one from the mother. The condition called VHL is caused by a dominant gene, since only one altered copy of the VHL gene will cause the condition. VHL occurs in both men and women. Each child of a person with VHL is at 50% risk of inheriting the altered copy of the gene.

The VHL gene is located on the short arm of chromosome 3 at a site called 3p25-p26. (see Figure 10.) An international team of scientists identified the precise structure of this gene in 1993. Alterations in the normal structure of this gene are known to result in the condition called VHL.

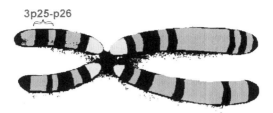

Figure 10: VHL gene location. The VHL gene is in the region 3p25-p26, near the tip of the short arm of chromosome 3. *Illustration by Karen Barnes, Stansbury Ronsaville Wood, Inc., for Howard Hughes Medical Institute, as published in Blazing a Genetic Trail, 1991*

The VHL gene encodes the formula for a protein whose function seems extremely important in the fundamental process called "transcription" which permits DNA to be transformed into a more simple molecule, RNA, which is used to create the protein.

The normal VHL gene acts as a "tumor-suppressor gene," whose normal function is to suppress the formation of tumors. In order for a tumor to form, both copies of the VHL gene (the one from the father and the one from the mother) must become inactivated. In an individual who does not have the inherited alteration in the VHL gene, it is necessary for each of these two normal copies of the VHL gene to undergo some change that inactivates the VHL protein and allows a tumor to form. This may take some time, and multiple damaging "hits" to the genes in this cell, before the tumor will form. This explains why when these tumors occur in the general population they are usually single occurrences in a single organ, and the average age of onset of symptomatic kidney cancer in the general population is age 62. Mutation or inactivation of the VHL gene has been found in 90% of the random clear cell kidney cancers in the general population studied by the U.S. National Cancer Institute (Linehan, *Nat Rev Urol*, 2010). This demonstrates the importance of this gene and the protein it manufactures in every human being.

In the case of people who have inherited one copy of the gene that doesn't work correctly in the beginning, it is only necessary to deactivate the one remaining copy before a tumor may form. This is a much more likely occurrence, which means that tumors develop more often, at younger ages, and in more organs than in people in the general population. Without preventive action, the average age of onset of symptomatic kidney cancer in people with VHL is age 42. (See Figure 11.)

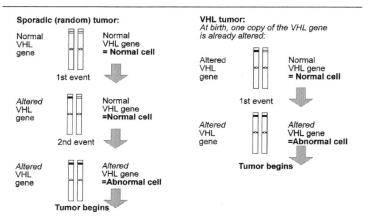

Figure 11: Path to development of a tumor. The VHL gene acts as a tumor suppressor gene. For a tumor to develop, both copies of the VHL gene (the one inherited from the father and the one inherited from the mother) must both become altered or otherwise inactivated. In people with VHL, one of these copies is already inactive, and only one additional step is required for a tumor to start. *Illustration from S. Richard and the French VHL.*

These alterations (or "mutations") of the VHL gene can now be identified in most people with VHL. The alteration is always the same in members of a single family. Conversely, the precise alteration in the gene will be different from one VHL family to another. More than 1548 individual mutations have already been described in the medical literature (Giles et al., *Human Mutat.* 2010). There is a significant relationship between certain kinds of mutations and the likelihood of pheochromocytomas, or the aggressiveness of Pancreatic NETs. Researchers are studying other specific mutations which may be responsible for different aspects of VHL.

In most cases, the alteration in the VHL gene occurred a very long time ago, and the original mutation has been passed down through several generations in a family. VHL in the Black Forest Family in Germany and Pennsylvania has been documented back to the early 1600's. There are certain people, though, perhaps as many as 20%, who are the first in their family to have an alteration in the VHL gene. Neither parent is affected, and these people have a case of VHL, occurring "*de novo*," for the first time. This "new mutation" is caused by a change in the gene in one sperm from the father, or in one egg from the mother, or in the copying of the gene in one of the first stages of division of the embryo. This alteration in the VHL gene can now be passed to future children of this affected person, and necessitates medical screening of these children as well. There are no reliable statistics yet on the rate of new VHL mutations.

Progress Toward a Cure

It is now possible to do special tests called DNA tests in most families to determine who does or does not carry the altered VHL gene. If you don't have the altered VHL gene, you cannot pass it to your children, and you need not go through further VHL screening tests. People who do not carry the gene can be reassured and spared further worry and testing. DNA testing methods are becoming less expensive and more accurate, and can now find the VHL gene alteration in most families. (See Section 6, *Obtaining DNA Testing*.)

With the gene identified, there is also increased hope of a cure, or at least of better management for VHL. Already in 2012 great strides have been made in improving diagnosis and treatment of VHL.

Scientists and the pharmaceutical companies are working to find a drug that will constrain tumor growth. As drugs are made available for clinical trials, announcements are posted in the *VHL Family Forum* and on the website, http://vhl.org.

> "The identification of tumor suppressor genes whose loss of function results in predisposition to cancer has taken center stage in our attempts to understand human carcinogenesis."
> — *Dr. Richard Klausner, then Chief, U.S. National Cancer Institute, 1995*

If VHL tumors can be kept small or made smaller, the amount of surgical intervention required to manage VHL can be minimized. Meanwhile our best defenses are "early detection and appropriate treatment." In the near term, knowledge and partnership with your healthcare team are your best defense.

Remember that the vast improvements in the survivability of prostate and breast cancer have been made without a curing drug—the most important advances have been in early detection and better treatment. The same can be said for VHL.

New research also shows that the VHL gene plays a role in a signaling system that tells the cell how much oxygen is available to it. When the VHL protein is missing, the cell believes—even if it is not true—that it is starving for oxygen. Its oxygen-sensing mechanism is broken. The cell puts out distress signals to the surrounding tissues, "Help! I need more oxygen!" Nearby blood vessels respond by building capillaries reaching toward the faulty cell to bring more blood to bring more oxygen. This response creates a mass of capillaries. Thus VHL tumors seem to be a normal self-protective response gone wrong. As we understand more about the function of the normal VHL protein, we have a better chance of finding a therapy that will fix or replace its function and keep tumors from growing.

In 1993 when the VHL gene was first discovered, the best description we had looked like this (see Figure 12):

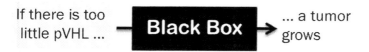

Figure 12: Black Box. All we knew in 1993 was that the VHL protein was essential to the healthy existence of the cell. When the protein was missing, its ability to regulate growth and replication was disrupted and cell growth went out of control.

Little by little, scientists have revealed more about the function of the VHL protein (pVHL) in the cell, and have found more "drug targets", or places where a drug might be used to change the outcome.

As part of its function, pVHL combines with other proteins in the cell. (see Figures 13 and 14.) Depending where the genetic alteration occurs, its ability to form connections with these other proteins may be impaired. We have learned a great deal about these differences by studying the relationship between the *genotype* (the place where the alteration occurs in the gene) and the *phenotype* (the set of symptoms experienced by these individuals).

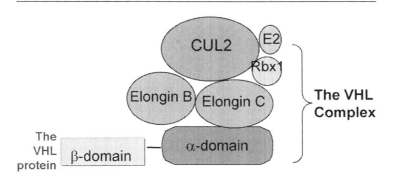

Figure 13: The VHL complex. The VHL protein (pVHL) combines with Elongins B and C and CUL2 to form a "complex", a kind of sub-assembly, which works as a machine to connect to other proteins in the cell and mark them for degradation and elimination — a kind of clean-up machine or "off" switch to stop processes from continuing. In this way it helps to control the levels of at least 17 other proteins in the cell. When this "off" function does not work properly, certain compounds are in over-supply and the process of cell growth and duplication goes out of control, resulting in a tumor or other malfunction. The alpha and beta domains marked are essentially connectors along pVHL that latch onto these other compounds. If the VHL mutation is in one of these connectors, the connector doesn't bind properly. *Source:* U.S. National Cancer Institute, *Science,* 269:1995, PNAS, 94:1997.

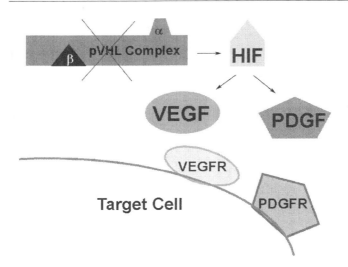

Figure 14: Pathways in the cell. If the pVHL complex is not functioning properly, then the levels of Hypoxia Inducible Factor (HIF) rise, which in turns allows the overproduction of Vascular Endothelial Growth Factor (VEGF) and Platelet-derived Growth Factor (PDGF) and others. These proteins send out signals to the target cell to stimulate the growth and reproduction of the cell. The signals are received by corresponding "receptors" (like VEGFR and PDGFR in this picture). In order to stop the signal from getting through, drugs may attempt to halt the signal, trap it in transit, or block the receptor. *Source:* W. G. Kaelin Jr., Dana-Farber Cancer Research Institute. *Clin Cancer Res.* 2004 Sep 15;10(18 Pt 2):6290S-5S.

Researchers have identified four categories of VHL, which may be useful in predicting the relative risk in a family for certain manifestations of VHL. These categories are not absolute; we still recommend screening for all the features of VHL, though the frequency of testing might be varied depending on the results of DNA testing. (See Table 2.) As time goes on and people with VHL are living longer, tumors may occur in a family where they have never been seen before. One family in France with more than 50 members in four generations had never experienced a pheo and was thought to be a Type 1 family. Recently, there have been pheos in two branches of that family. Similarly, families thought to be Type 2A have found that as they reach their 50's for the first time, several are developing kidney cancer. These classifications are useful to the researchers, but so far have limited usefulness in the clinic.

Table 2: Genotype-phenotype classifications in families with von Hippel-Lindau disease*.
Source: Lancet 2003; 361: 2062.

	Clinical Characteristics
Type 1	Retinal hemangioblastomas CNS hemangioblastomas Renal cell carcinoma Pancreatic tumors and cysts
Type 2A	Pheochromocytomas Retinal hemangioblastomas CNS hemangioblastomas
Type 2B	Pheochromocytomas Retinal hemangioblastomas CNS hemangioblastomas Renal cell carcinomas Pancreatic tumors and cysts
Type 2C	Pheochromocytoma only

*Endolymphatic sac tumors and cystadenomas of the epididymis and broad ligament have not been assigned to specific von Hippel-Lindau types.

Much has been learned about pVHL from the study of other diseases in the same general disease area, such as the many genetic flaws that can lead to a pheochromocytoma or kidney cancer. (See Figure 15.) In fact, the body is an elegant system of sensors and controls and backup systems. More than one path is provided to ensure that essential functions are carried out reliably. VHL may be on one path, but there is frequently a second or third path that serves as a backup.

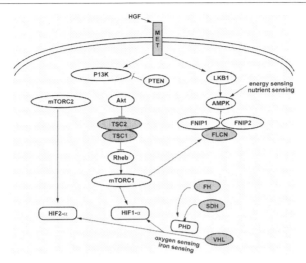

Figure 15: The genetics of kidney cancer. This diagram shows the kidney cancer pathways. Notice that on this one map we can see the genes responsible for the seven known genetic causes of kidney cancer: VHL, FH (for HLRCC), FLCN (for BHD), TSC1 & 2 (for TS), MET (for HPRCC) and SDH (for SDHB & D). Linehan et al., "The genetic basis of kidney cancer: a metabolic disease," *Nat Rev Urol* 2010 May:7(5):277-85.

Most are also multi-function controls — they not only turn on one feature, they may have the ability to control a large number of functions. For example, we now know that pVHL not only influences angiogenesis, it also plays a role in oxygen sensing, iron sensing, and the metabolism of glucose (glycolysis).

At this time in 2012 there are six new drugs on the market approved for "advanced"(metastatic) kidney cancer, based in large part on research on the VHL gene and its protein product, pVHL:

- Bevacizumab (Avastin)
- Sunitinib (Sutent)
- Sorafenib (Nexavar)
- Everolimus (Afinitor)
- Temsirolimus (Torisel)
- Pazopanib (Votrient)

There have been some limited trials of these drugs for VHL. So far the kidney and pancreas tumors show limited response to these drugs, and the brain and spinal tumors show almost no response. As of 2012 the trial of pazopanib for VHL is only beginning. More drugs will be coming on the market, targeting different points on the signaling shown on these pathways—inhibiting the production of a protein, or inhibiting the ability of its "receptor" to receive its signal. As these drugs are developed further, it is expected that their next generations will be more "specific" (go directly to the right spot and do the job more effectively) and will have fewer side effects.

Perhaps some day it will be possible to replace pVHL chemically. Injecting it into the bloodstream does not help; it has to be put deep into the cell. Some experimental methods in the areas of gene therapy, nanotechnology or stem cell therapy may permit replacement or correction of the genetic information. These technologies are still in their infancy. Success in using these technologies for any one disease may provide an exciting mechanism for VHL as well.

Promoting Research and Clinical Trials

You and your family can help to move the progress of VHL research forward by contributing samples of blood and tumor tissue to any local research projects you can. See http://vhl.org/bank for information about tissue banking.

For example, there are a number of efforts to identify biomarkers. These markers, found in blood or urine, would indicate the level of tumor activity in the body without expensive scans. In order to find such biomarkers, researchers need samples of blood and urine from a large number of people with VHL. Please help whenever you can.

Tissue from VHL tumors is needed to test potential therapies in the lab and determine what might be a good candidate for a clinical trial. When surgery is planned, call the VHL Tissue Bank and register to donate the tissue your surgeon will be removing. The Bank will arrange for tissue collection with your surgeon. Ideally, tissue should be flash frozen in the operating room itself. Tissue not recovered within 24 hours cannot be used for research. (See Section 10, *Tissue Bank,* for the donor registration form.)

When clinical trials are announced, please read the announcement to determine whether the drug offered might be appropriate to your particular circumstances. Please consider participating in trials when they are right for you. Your top priority should always be to do what is best for your present and long-term health.

News of the current state of VHL research and clinical trials is carried in the *VHL Family Forum*.

The VHL Family Alliance works to encourage research on von Hippel-Lindau through the Research Database, the VHL Tissue Bank, the VHL Fund for Cancer Research, and the VHLFA Research Grants program. (See *Support our Efforts!* at the end of this book.) Please help to sustain these efforts.

References:

Frew, IK, Krek W, Multitasking by pVHL in tumour suppression, *Curr Opin Cell Biol,* 2007 Dec:19(6):685-90, PMID: 18006292

Kaelin WG Jr, The von Hippel-Lindau tumor suppressor gene and kidney cancer, *Clin Cancer Res.* 2004 Sep 15;10(18 Pt 2):6290S-5S. PMID: 15448019

Kaelin, WG Jr, Role of VHL gene mutation in human cancer, *J Clin Oncol.* 2004 Dec 15;22(24):4991-5004., PMID: 15611513

Kaelin, WG Jr, von Hippel-Lindau disease. *Annu Rev Pathol.* 2007;2:145-73. PMID: 18039096

Kaelin, WG Jr, Treatment of kidney cancer: insights provided by the VHL tumor-suppressor protein, *Cancer.* 2009 May 15;115(10 Suppl):2262-72, PMID: 19402056

Latif F, et al., Identification of the von Hippel-Lindau Disease Tumor Suppressor Gene. *Science.* 1993 260:1317-1320. PMID: 8493574

Li L, et al., New insights into the biology of renal cell carcinoma, *Hematol Oncol Clin North Am.* 2011 Aug; 25(4):667-86. PMID: 21763962

Linehan WM, et al., Molecular diagnosis and therapy of kidney cancer, *Annu Rev Med.* 2010; 61:329-43. PMID: 20059341; Nat Rev Urol. 2010 May;7(5):277-85. PMID: 20059341

Linehan WM, Srinivasan R, Schmidt LS, The genetic basis of kidney cancer: a metabolic disease. *Nat Rev Urol.* 2010 May;7(5):277-85., PMID: 20448661

Nordstrong-O'Brien M., Giles R, et al., Genetic analysis of von Hippel-Lindau disease. *Hum Mutat.* 2010 May;31(50):521-37. PMID: 20151405

Shen C, Kaelin WG, et al., Genetic and Functional Studies Implicate HIF 1a as a 14q Kidney Cancer Suppressor Gene, *Cancer Discov.* 2011 Aug;1(3):222-235., PMID: 22037472

Tsuchiva MI, Shuin T, et al., Renal cell carcinoma- and pheochromocytoma-specific altered gene expression profiles in VHL mutant clones, *Oncol Rep.* 2005 Jun;13(6):1033-41., PMID: 15870918

Section 4:
Living Well with VHL

There is no magic pill—yet!—that will make VHL go away. VHL is a lifelong challenge. It is less demanding of your attention than something like diabetes—you don't have to check your blood sugar multiple times a day or change every aspect of your diet—but you do need to put the right level of attention onto monitoring it, keeping your mind, body, and spirit strong, and keeping this issue in perspective in the whole of your life.

It is important to take care of your general level of health. If you make sure that you are in good health, then the challenges VHL throws your way will be easier to meet. Eat right, don't smoke, exercise, drive carefully, and don't hide behind alcohol or drugs. Eat less red meat, and eat a diet based more on vegetable sources. (see Figure 16.) Watch for cancer-prevention tips in the press for ideas on how to keep your body's own natural defenses strong against the forces that promote cancer by causing genes to become deactivated. This area is being closely studied, and reliable information is emerging, especially from the work of the American Institute for Cancer Research (AICR), the World Cancer Research Fund (WCRF), and the Harvard School of Public Health.

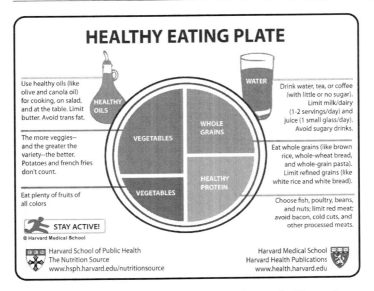

Figure 16: Health Eating Plate. *Source:* Willett et al., Harvard School of Public Health, 2011.

One of the greatest known risk factors for any medical condition is smoking. Studies on kidney tumors in the general population indicate that patients who smoke, especially men, have more tumors than those who don't, and that those tumors grow more rapidly. People who smoke are at higher risk for a number of post-operative complications.

There is no evidence to indicate that VHL patients should limit their physical activities in any way, except for short periods following treatments. Certain kinds of brain, spinal, or eye tumors may be aggravated by doing a lot of heavy straining: bench-pressing 200 pound weights so that the veins in your forehead stand out, pumping your exercising heart rate beyond your recommended limits, or going through the hardest parts of labor in childbirth. Check with your doctor to determine your own exercise tolerance. Moderate exercise, however, is good for everyone.

In brief: eat smart and move more. The three key factors recommended by AICR and WCRF are:

1. Eat a diet based primarily on plant foods rather than animal sources.

2. Limit red meat, and avoid processed meats (sausage, bacon).
3. Be physically active within everyday life. Stop gaining weight; eat healthy to achieve and maintain a healthy body weight.

In addition, research is showing that more than one-third of the population in the United States and other developed countries is deficient in Vitamin D. Vitamin D is important to keep our immune systems strong, and for bone health. People with reduced kidney function are particularly prone to Vitamin D deficiency. While our bodies normally make Vitamin D when exposed to sun, we are living more of our lives indoors than ever before. Kidney and pancreas issues can interfere with Vitamin D absorbtion. There is a simple blood test for Vitamin D which many doctors have already added to their routine blood testing. Ask what your levels are, and take Vitamin D3 supplements to get your levels to at least 50 (60–70 preferred).

> "One of the most important fields of medical science over the past 50 years is the research that shows just how powerfully our health is affected by what we eat. Knowing what foods to eat and in what proportions is crucial for health. The evidence-based Healthy Eating Plate shows this is a way that is very simple to understand."
> – *Anthony Komaroff, Professor of Medicine at Harvard Medical School and Editor in Chief of Harvard Health Publications, 2011.*

There is growing evidence that prolonged inflammation may have some influence on the course of diseases such as cancer, Alzheimer's and heart disease. Dr. Weil recommends a diet rich in omega-3 fatty acids (extra-virgin olive oil, expeller-pressed canola oil, nuts — especially walnuts, avocados and seeds — hemp seeds, freshly ground flaxseed and oily fishes are good sources). Use natural anti-inflammatory spices like garlic, ginger, turmeric and cinnamon. Vitamin D3 also helps to control inflammation.

VHL is a chronic disease, a lifelong challenge. While it may not affect your life on a day-to-day basis, every once in a while it will jump into first place, demanding your attention. If you work with your medical team to monitor it on a regular basis, you will be able to maintain greater control over the situation and manage the interruptions that it may cause in your life. By keeping up with a regular program of medical check-ups, you can reduce your worry of the unknown.

References:

Food, Nutrition, Physical Activity and the Prevention of Cancer: a global perspective, 1997, 2007.
  http://www.dietandcancerreport.org/
AICR video summary of this report:
  http://www.vimeo.com/21464219
Healthy Eating Plate, from the Harvard School of Public Health. See http://www.health.harvard.edu/plate/healthy-eating-plate
Diet, Nutrition, and Cancer Prevention: The Good News, U.S. National Institutes of Health, various publications are available from 1-800-4CANCER
Campbell, T. Colin, *The China Study*, 2006
Wu S., Sun J, Vitamin D, Vitamin D receptor, and macroautophagy in inflammation and infection. *Discov Med.* 2011 Apr;11(59):325-35. PMID: 21524386
Dyck, et al., The anticancer efffects of Vitamin D and omega-3 PUFAs in combination via cod-liver oil: One plus one may equal more than two. *Med Hypotheses.* 2011 May 30. PMID: 21632182

The Healthy Eating Plate

The Healthy Eating Plate from the Harvard School of Public Health incorporates new learning about nutrition and cancer prevention. The Healthy Eating Plate sits on a foundation of daily exercise and weight control. Why? These two related elements strongly influence your chances of staying healthy. They also affect what and how you eat and how your food affects you. The other bricks of the Healthy Eating Plate include:

Whole Grain Foods (at most meals). The body needs carbohydrates mainly for energy. The best sources of carbohydrates are whole grains such as oatmeal, whole-wheat bread, and brown rice. They deliver the outer (bran) and inner (germ) layers along with energy-rich starch. The body can't digest whole grains as quickly as it can highly processed carbohydrates such as white flour. This keeps blood sugar and insulin levels from rising, then falling, too quickly. Better control of blood sugar and insulin can keep hunger at bay and may prevent the development of type 2 diabetes.

Plant Oils. The bottle of oil next to the Healthy Eating Plate shows the importance of healthy fats. Note, that it specifically mentions plant oils, not all types of fat. Good sources of healthy unsaturated fats include extra-virgin olive oil, canola, and other plant oils, as well as fatty fish such as salmon. These healthy fats not only improve cholesterol levels (when eaten in place of highly processed carbohydrates) but can also protect the heart from sudden and potentially deadly rhythm problems. Limit butter and trans fat.

Vegetables (in abundance). A diet rich in fruits and vegetables can decrease the chances of having a heart attack or stroke; protect against a variety of cancers; lower blood pressure; help you avoid the painful intestinal ailment called diverticulitis; guard against cataract and macular degeneration; and add variety to your diet and wake up your palate. Limit consumption of potatoes, which has the same roller-coaster effect on blood sugar as refined grains and sweets.

Fruits (2 to 3 times daily): Choose a rainbow of fruits every day: fresh in season or frozen, organic when possible.

Healthy Proteins: Choose fish, poultry, beans or nuts, which contain healthful nutrients. A wealth of research suggests that eating fish can reduce the risk of heart disease. Chicken and turkey are also good sources of protein and can be low in saturated fat. Limit red meat and avoid processed meats, since eating even small quantities of these on a regular basis raises the risk of heart disease, type 2 diabetes, colon cancer, and weight gain. Eggs, which have long been demonized because they contain fairly high levels of cholesterol, aren't as bad as they're cracked up to be. In fact, an egg is a much better breakfast than a doughnut cooked in an oil rich in trans fats or a bagel made from refined flour. Nuts and legumes are excellent sources of protein, fiber, vitamins, and minerals. Legumes include black beans, navy beans, garbanzos, and other beans that are usually sold dried. Many kinds of nuts contain healthy fats, and packages of some varieties (almonds, walnuts, pecans, peanuts, hazelnuts, and pistachios) even carry a label saying they're good for your heart.

Water, juice, and dairy: Drink water, tea, or coffee (with little or no sugar). Limit milk and dairy (1–2 servings per day) and juice (1 small glass a day) and avoid sugary drinks. Building bone and keeping it strong takes calcium, vitamin D, exercise, and a whole lot more. Dairy products have traditionally been the main source of calcium. But there is also a lot of fat in whole milk and cheese. Three glasses of whole milk, for example, contains as much saturated fat as 13 strips of cooked bacon. If you enjoy dairy foods, try to stick with no fat or low fat products. If you don't like dairy products, calcium supplements offer an easy and inexpensive way to get your daily calcium.

Multiple vitamin: A daily multivitamin, multimineral supplement offers a kind of nutritional backup. While it cannot in any way replace healthy eating, or make up for unhealthy eating, it can fill in the nutrient holes that may sometimes affect even the most careful eaters. You do not need an expensive name-brand or designer vitamin. A standard, store-brand, RDA-level one is fine. Look for one that meets the requirements of the USP (U.S. Pharmacopeia), or another organization that sets standards for drugs and supplements.

Use alcohol in moderation: Scores of studies suggest that having an alcoholic drink a day lowers the risk of heart disease. Moderation is clearly important, since alcohol has risks as well as benefits. For men, a good balance point is 1 to 2 drinks a day. For women, it's at most one drink a day.

Harvard Healthy Eating Plate and discussion adapted from Willett, Eat, Drink, and Be Healthy, Harvard School of Public Health, 2001, 2008, 2011

Living with Knowing

Having a chronic disease is a stressful experience. It is easy to say you should think of a brain tumor as a wart, but it is easier said than done. No one can completely avoid stress; it is an essential part of living. Consider incorporating into your life a stress management program that works for you. There are many different kinds—sports, yoga, prayer, meditation—it does not matter which one you choose as long as you do it. (See Figure 17.)

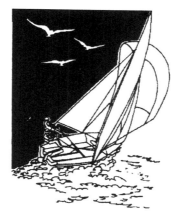

Figure 17: The Art of Conscious Living. "When we are able to mobilize our inner resources to face our problems artfully, we find we are usually able to orient ourselves in such a way that we can use the pressure of the problem itself to propel us through it, just as a sailor can position a sail to make the best use of the pressure of the wind to propel the boat. You can't sail straight into the wind, and if you only know how to sail with the wind at your back, you will only go where the wind blows you. But if you know how to use the wind energy and are patient you can sometimes get where you want to go. You can still be in control… We all accept that no one controls the weather. Good sailors learn to read it carefully and respect its power. They will avoid storms if possible, but when caught in one, they know when to take down the sails, batten down the hatches, drop anchor, and ride things out, controlling what is controllable and letting go of the rest… Developing skill in facing and effectively handling the various "weather conditions" in your life is what we mean by the art of conscious living."
— *Jon Kabat-Zinn, Ph.D., Director of the Stress Reduction Clinic at the University of Massachusetts Medical Center, Worcester, Massachusetts. As quoted from his book,* Full Catastrophe Living: Using the Wisdom of your Body and Mind to Face Stress, Pain and Illness, *p. 3. (Delta Books, New York, 1990, 2009).*

Pay attention to stress management on a regular basis. Scientific research has produced well-documented and conclusive data verifying the benefits of regular meditation practice and various mind/body approaches to stress reduction and improving emotional and physical health. Most major medical centers now have stress reduction programs. These approaches can have a profound healing effect on the entire person—emotionally, intellectually, physically, socially, and spiritually. Ask your medical team for a referral to a stress management program, or visit your local bookstore and find a book that you feel will be meaningful to you. Consider one by Benson, Kabat-Zinn, Borysenko, David Burns, Albert Ellis, or another of the many physicians whose stress-reduction programs have been shown to soften the course of chronic illness. The VHL Family Alliance maintains a list of suggested readings on stress management that have been found to be medically beneficial. (See *Some Suggestions for Reading*, below.)

Assertiveness training can help you reduce your anxiety and improve your effectiveness in dealing with doctors and complex situations.

A chronic disease can put strain on the best of marriages. Don't be shy to ask for help or counseling. You are not alone. It is not your fault. VHL is not a punishment; it is a disease.

Husbands, wives, parents, and children will all feel the strain in different ways. Affected people have the very real mental and physical pressures of the disease and its treatments and effects. It is normal to go through denial, anger, and a whole range of fragile emotions. It is normal to feel more needful, and to be angry when your family does not automatically understand your needs. It is important to talk with your family about how you are feeling. You are not burdening them; you are giving them the privilege of participating with you. It is less stressful on everyone when you are partners in dealing with VHL.

Unaffected members of the family will feel their own strains, anger and guilt. Unaffected children may be angry that the affected child gets all the attention, or may feel guilty that they were spared. Affected or not, children often harbor unspoken fears for themselves or for their parents, which may come out as misbehavior or school performance issues. Schools often have social workers or psychologists who can be called upon to assist children. In some areas there are support groups for children whose families are affected by cancer or chronic illness.

Finding out you have VHL is a traumatic event, which quite naturally results in unpleasant reactions. It is normal to feel anger, and it is important to work through those feelings to reach a place where you can turn that negative energy into constructive action to protect yourself and others in your family.

With patience, understanding, and the assistance of your medical and spiritual advisers and friends, your family will survive this challenge and thrive.

Family Support

It also helps to talk with someone who is on the same journey. Join a family support program, such as the VHL Family Alliance. Pick up the phone and call, if only just to talk for a while, or join the online support group. Other families with VHL are there to listen and to share their own experiences, which may help you gain a different perspective on the problem. Listen and learn, or join in the conversation. Participate in local support group meetings.

Think of it as an old-fashioned barn-raising. (see Figure 18.) One person, even one couple, can't raise a barn alone. The community, though, can come together and do it in a few days, pooling skills and experiences and making the task easier. Each member of the group benefits in turn from the community effort.

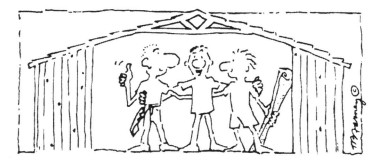

Figure 18: "Self-help is barn raising revisited." – Len Borman, founder, Illinois Self-Help Center. As quoted in Power Tools: Ways to Build a Self-Help Group by Joal Fischer, M.D. *Art by Tina B. Farney. Booklet and art copyright 1992 by SupportWorks, Charlotte, North Carolina. All rights reserved. Reprinted with the kind permission of Ms. Farney and Dr. Fischer.*

It can be frightening to reach out, but it is much worse to be alone. Besides, *we* need to hear from *you*. It is through sharing information that this organization was born. It is through putting our shared experience and information together with the expertise of the caring physicians and researchers who are also working on VHL, that we are learning the keys to improving diagnosis, treatment, and quality of life for everyone with VHL.

> "Bringing people together by building on personal relationships remains one of the most effective strategies to enhance America's social health."
> — *Robert D. Putnam, Better Together*

Talking with Children about VHL

Children who have a DNA diagnosis of VHL will begin to have questions about VHL, sometimes at early ages. The VHL Family Alliance has prepared a book for children about VHL, to assist parents in having a constructive conversation about what this diagnosis means to the child, and what the child can do to help stay healthy. Please see the *VHL Handbook, Kids' Edition (2009) by Kruger, Eckerman, Doyle, and Chan-Smutko. ISBN 978-1-929539-02-4* Available through internet bookstores or at vhl.org.

This *Kids' Handbook* is written specifically as a guide to help you talk with children about von Hippel-Lindau, a hereditary cancer syndrome that increases one's risk of having tumors of the eye, brain, spinal cord, kidneys, pancreas, and adrenal glands. It is meant to give children of all ages a basic idea about VHL and how we can use this information to manage out health.

The book can also be used as a starting point for discussions about how VHL has affected the family. It may be helpful for families dealing with any hereditary cancer syndrome. The book may be most helpful when a member of the family has been directly affected, and your children may be facing testing themselves.

Written and reviewed by a team of parents and professionals, and illustrated with charming drawings and photographs from children with VHL, their siblings and friends, the book is upbeat and hopeful, helping children understand what is happening, and learn to share responsibility for managing their health.

Some Suggestions for Reading

Robert E. Alberti, et al., *Your Perfect Right: Assertiveness and Equality in your Life and Relationships* (9th edition, 2008)

Herbert Benson, M.D., *Timeless Healing: The Power and Biology of Belief* (1996)

Joan Borysenko, Ph.D., *Minding the Body, Mending the Mind* (1987)

Jeffrey Brantley, M.D., *Calming the Anxious Mind* (2007)

David Burns, *Feeling Good: The New Mood Therapy* (1999)

David Burns, *Feeling Good Together* (2010)

Albert Ellis, *Feeling Better, Getting Better, Staying Better* (2001)

John A. Gottman, Ph.D. and Jean DeClaire, *The Relationship Cure* (2001)

Jerome Groopman, M.D., *The Anatomy of Hope: How People Prevail in the Face of Illness* (2003)

Jerome Groopman, *Second Opinions: Stories of Intuition and Choice in the Changing World of Medicine* (2000)

Jon Kabat-Zinn, *Full Catastrophe Living: Using the Wisdom of your Body and Mind to Face Stress, Pain, and Illness* (1990, 2009)

Harold S. Kushner, *When Bad Things Happen to Good People* (1981)

Harold S. Kushner, *Overcoming Life's Disappointments* (2007); *Conquering Fear* (2010)

Robert D. Putnam, *Better Together: Restoring the American Community* (2005, 2009)

McCue, Kathleen, and Ron Bonn, *How to Help Children Through a Parent's Serious Illness* (1994)

Questions to Ask the Doctor

With early detection and appropriate treatment, von Hippel-Lindau disease has a better prognosis, or outcome, than many other tumor conditions and cancers. But any diagnosis of serious illness can be frightening. It is natural to have concerns about medical tests, treatments, insurance, and doctors' bills.

Patients have many important questions to ask about VHL, and their medical team is the best place to start to look for answers. Most people want to know exactly what kind of involvement they have, how it can be treated, and how successful the treatment is likely to be. Get a second,

or even a third opinion if you wish. The following are some questions that patients may want to ask their physician:
- Should I change my normal activities?
- How often are checkups needed?
- What symptoms should I watch for?
- If you are told what size a tumor is (e.g., 2 cm.), ask what that means.
- At what point do I need to worry about this tumor?
- What are the danger signals we are watching for?
- What kinds of treatment are available?
- What are the risks or side effects of treatment?
- What are the odds of those risks happening?
- What are the risks of no treatment?
- Is there a less invasive treatment I should consider?
- Can abdominal surgery be done laparoscopically?
- What other health professionals do I need on my medical team to ensure that we have checked for all the probable features of VHL?
- What can I do to assist doctors in learning more about VHL?
- How experienced are you in dealing with VHL?
- Where can I consult specialists who are experienced with VHL?
- Who will be the main person responsible for looking after my medical interests and coordinating communication among my specialists?
- Is there a research project in which I can participate?
- Is there a clinical trial that would be appropriate for me?

The VHL Athlete

"In preparing myself for a delicate spinal surgery, I was naturally not looking forward to the experience, but knew that I had to get through it if I wanted to alleviate the growing numbness and have use of my arms and hands. I looked for a good role model. I noticed that marathon runners, or competitors in triathalons, also push themselves up to and beyond their physical limits. They endure pain, thirst, and suffering, all to win the prize, to compete sometimes more with themselves than with the others in the race.

In addition to the careful preparation my doctors and I went through, consulting with specialists throughout the world to choose the best approaches for the surgery, I trained myself for this even as if I were training for a sports event. I made sure my body was healthy and strong, tuned with vitamins and healthy natural foods, and that my mind was strong as well. Through meditation and guided imagery, I pictured the surgery going well, the surgeons confident and successful, and my body helping to minimize bleeding and recover quickly. I worked with a sports trainer and used sports psychology.

The day of the surgery arrived, and our team—my doctors and I—worked through the day. By evening, I was awake, squeezing my husband Bruce's hand and wiggling my toes. Everyone cheered. We had won the first event in the triathalon—now on to physical therapy and back to normal life."

— *Jennifer K., Australia*

Reminder Calendar

Next Check-Ups

Date	Doctor	Tests	Results	Return Date

See also the "Care Booklet" available at http://vhl.org

Section 5:
Suggested Screening Guidelines

Screening is the testing of individuals at risk for von Hippel-Lindau disease (VHL) who do not yet have symptoms, or who are known to have VHL but do not yet have symptoms in a particular area. The unaffected organs should still be screened.

Modifications of screening schedules may sometimes be done by physicians familiar with individual patients and with their family history. Once a person has a known manifestation of VHL, or develops a symptom, the follow-up plan should be determined with the medical team. More frequent testing may be needed to track the growth of known lesions.

People who have had a DNA test and do not carry the altered VHL gene may be excused from testing. Even with the VHL gene, once an individual has reached the age of sixty and still has no evidence of VHL on these screening tests, imaging tests may be every two years for MRI.

Revisions in this version of the screening protocol include a change in recommendations from CT to MRI, in order to reduce exposure to radiation for all people. CT should be avoided for all pre-symptomatic people, and should be reserved for occasions when it is truly needed to answer a diagnostic question.

In order to monitor the most critical areas of the brain and spinal cord in the most efficient and cost-effective manner, it is recommended to order an "MRI with contrast of brain and cervical spine, with thin cuts through the posterior fossa, and attention to inner ear/petrous temporal bone to rule out both ELST and hemangioblastomas of neuraxis".

Regular audiometric tests are included in the screening protocol to provide a reference point in case of sign or symptom of hearing loss, tinnitus (ringing in the ears), and/or vertigo (dizziness, loss of balance). If hearing drops, swift action may be required to save hearing. The Danish group is heading a study of audiometric information to determine whether early signs of ELST might be detected. Your participation will be appreciated. Write to info@vhl.org.

MRI is the preferred screening method for the abdomen. Quality ultrasound may be substituted for MRI of the abdomen no more than once every two years. "Quality" is defined as a machine that produces good quality pictures, with an operator experienced in imaging the organs being studied. The objective is to find even small tumors, which are difficult to identify on ultrasound.

Any Age
- Inform families that, if they choose, they and their geneticist may contact one of the clinical DNA testing laboratories familiar with VHL for DNA testing. If the family marker is detectable, DNA testing can identify those family members who are not at risk and may discontinue screening. Testing may also be useful in calculating risks for family members who do carry the altered gene and require periodic screening tests. Risk factors are not definitive indicators of what will happen, but only highlight areas at higher or lower risk probability. Early detection and appropriate treatment are our best defenses.

From Conception
- Inform obstetrician of family history of VHL. If the mother has VHL, see also the discussion of pregnancy in this booklet and in the screening protocol. A mother-to-be who is having any genetic testing done may request a VHL test be included in that series of tests.

From Birth
- Inform pediatrician of family history of VHL. Pediatrician to look for signs of neurological disturbance, nystagmus, strabismus, white pupil, and other signs which might indicate a referral to a retinal specialist. Routine newborn hearing screening.

Age 1–4
Annually:
- Eye/retinal examination with indirect ophthalmoscope by ophthalmologist skilled in diagnosis & management

of retinal disease, especially for children known to carry the VHL mutation.
- Pediatrician to look for signs of neurological disturbance, nystagmus, strabismus, white pupil, and abnormalities in blood pressure, vision, or hearing.

Ages 5–15
Annually:
- Physical examination and neurological assessment by pediatrician informed about VHL, with particular attention to blood pressure, lying and standing, hearing issues, neurological disturbance, nystagmus, strabismus, white pupil, and other signs which might indicate a referral to a retinal specialist.
- Eye/retinal examination with indirect ophthalmoscope by ophthalmologist informed about VHL, using a dilated exam.
- Test for fractionated metanephrines, especially normetanephrine in a "plasma free normetanephrine" blood test or in a 24-hour urine test. Abdominal ultrasonography annually from 8 years or earlier if indicated. Abdominal MRI or MIBG scan only if biochemical abnormalities found.

Every 2–3 years:
- Complete audiology assessment by an audiologist. Annually if any hearing loss, tinnitus, or vertigo is found.
- In the case of repeated ear infections, MRI with contrast of the internal auditory canal using thin slices, to check for a possible ELST.

Age 16 and beyond
Annually:
- Eye/retinal examination with indirect ophthalmoscope by ophthalmologist informed about VHL, using a dilated exam.
- Quality ultrasound, and at least every other year MRI scan of abdomen with and without contrast to assess kidneys, pancreas, adrenals, but *not* during pregnancy. Physical examination by physician informed about VHL.

- Test for fractionated metanephrines, especially normetanephrine in "plasma free metanephrines" blood test or 24-hour urine test. Abdominal MRI or MIBG scan if biochemical abnormalities found.

Every two years:
- "MRI with contrast of brain and cervical spine, with thin cuts through the posterior fossa, and attention to inner ear/petrous temporal bone to rule out both ELST and hemangioblastomas of neuraxis"
- Audiology assessment by an audiologist.

During pregnancy
- Regular retinal checkup to anticipate potentially more rapid progression of lesions
- Test for pheo early, mid, and again late pregnancy to ensure no active pheo during pregnancy or especially labor and delivery.
- During the 4th month of pregnancy, MRI — without contrast — to check on any known lesions of the brain and spine. If known retinal, brain, or spinal lesions, consider C-section.

References:

Maher ER, Neumann HP, Richard S., von Hippel-Lindau disease: a clinical and scientific review. *Eur J Hum Genet.* 2011 Jun;19(6):617-23. Epub 2011 Mar 9. PMID: 21386872

Richard S, Lindau J, Graff J, Resche F. Von Hippel-Lindau disease. *Lancet*, 2004, 363: 1231-4. PMID: 15081659

Lonser RR, Glenn GM, Chew EY, Libutti SK, Linehan WM, Oldfield EH, von Hippel-Lindau disease. *Lancet.* 2003 Jun 14;361(9374):2059-67. PMID: 12814730

Commonly Occurring VHL Manifestations

Age at onset varies from family to family and from individual to individual. The figures shown in Table 3 include age at symptomatic diagnosis, particularly in the early literature, and age at presymptomatic diagnosis because of a screening protocol. With better diagnostic techniques, diagnoses are being made earlier. This does not mean that action needs to be taken when early lesions are found, but care must be taken to watch the progression of these lesions and act at the appropriate moment.

Pheochromocytoma is very common in some families, while renal cell carcinoma is more common in other families. Individuals in a family may differ as to which of the family tumor types they express.

Pancreatic neuroendocrine tumors may be more aggressive in people with an alteration in exon 3.

Rare manifestations include cerebral (upper brain) hemangioblastoma, and rare occurrences of hemangioma in liver, spleen and lung.

Table 3: Occurrence and age of onset in VHL.
Compiled from a survey of papers from 1976 through 2004, and including data from the VHL Family Alliance.

	Ages at Diagnosis	Most common ages at dx	Frequency in patients
CNS			
Retinal hemangioblastomas	0–68 yrs	12–25 yrs	25–60%
Endolymphatic sac tumors	12–46 yrs	24–35 yrs	10–25%
Cerebellar hemangioblastomas	9–78 yrs	18–25 yrs	44–72%
Brainstem hemangioblastomas	12–36 yrs	24–35 yrs	10–25%
Spinal cord hemangioblastomas	12–66 yrs	24–35 yrs	13–50%
Viscera			
Renal cell carcinoma or cysts	16–67 yrs	25–50 yrs	25–60%
Pheochromocytomas*	4–58 yrs	12–25 yrs	10–20%**
Pancreatic tumor or cyst	5–70 yrs	24–35 yrs	35–70%
Epididymal cystadenomas	17–43 yrs	14–40 yrs	25–60% of males
APMO or broad ligament cystadenomas	16–64 yrs	16–46 yrs	est. 10% of females

* Includes the 20% of these tumors that occur outside the adrenal gland, also called paragangliomas.
** Frequency of pheochromocytoma varies widely depending on genotype. Refer to Table 2.

Common Treatment Recommendations

There are no universal treatment recommendations; treatment options can only be determined by careful evaluation of the patient's total situation: symptoms, test results, imaging studies, and general physical condition. The following are offered as general guidelines for possible treatment therapies. Doctors are asked to read Lonser et al., (*Lancet*, 2003; 361:2059-67) for a more detailed explanation.

Retinal angiomas: In the periphery, consider treatment of small lesions with laser and larger lesions with cryotherapy. If the angioma is on the optic disc, follow the growth pattern. There are few treatment options for tumors of the optic disc. The optimal treatment would be a drug, but to date none has proven successful. Check with one of the expert centers for the latest treatment options for angiomas on or near the optic nerve.

Brain and spinal hemangioblastomas: Symptoms related to hemangioblastomas in the brain and spinal cord depend on tumor location and size, and the presence of associated swelling or cysts. Symptomatic lesions grow more rapidly than asymptomatic lesions. Cysts often cause more symptoms than the tumor itself. Once the lesion has been removed, the cyst will collapse. If any portion of the tumor is left in place, the cyst will re-fill. Small hemangioblastomas (under 3 cubic cm, or 1.7 cm measured diagonally) which are not symptomatic and are not associated with a cyst have sometimes been treated with stereotactic radiosurgery, but this is more a preventive than a treatment, and long-term results seem to show only marginal benefit. (Asthagiri, *Neuro Oncology*, 2010.)

Endolymphatic sac tumors: Patients who have a tumor or hemorrhage visible on MRI but who can still hear require surgery to prevent a worsening of their condition. Deaf patients with evidence on imaging of a tumor should undergo surgery if other neurological symptoms are present, in order to prevent worsening of balance problems. Further study is needed to determine whether patients with clinical symptoms of ELST, but without evidence of a tumor or hemorrhage on imaging, should undergo surgery to prevent hearing loss or to alleviate symptoms. (Lonser et al., *J Neurosurgery*, 2008)

Pheochromocytoma: Surgery after adequate blocking with medication. Laparoscopic partial adrenalectomy is preferred. Careful monitoring of vital signs for at least a week following surgery, as the body readjusts to its "new normal." Special caution is warranted during surgical procedures of any type, and during pregnancy and delivery. There is a debate over the wisdom of leaving in place pheos which do not appear to be active and are not causing symptoms. US NIH generally monitors small pheos until urinary catecholamines are at least two times the upper limit of normal (even if plasma catecholamines are elevated).

Renal Cell Carcinoma: With improved imaging techniques, kidney tumors are often found at very small sizes, and at very early stages of development. A strategy for insuring that an individual will have sufficient functioning kidney throughout his or her lifetime begins with careful monitoring and choosing to operate only when tumor size or rapid growth rate suggest the tumor may gain metastatic potential (approximately 3 cm). The technique of kidney sparing surgery is widely used in this setting. *Radio Frequency Ablation* (RFA) or cryotherapy may be considered, especially for smaller tumors at earlier stages, though care must be taken not to injure adjacent structures, and to limit scarring which may complicate subsequent surgeries. Robotic surgery can be used to limit scarring (Matin et al., *BJU Int*, 2008, and Hoeffel et al., *Euro Radiol,* 2010 and Gupta et al., *Urol Oncology*, 2011)

Pancreatic Neuroendocrine Tumors: Careful analysis is required to differentiate between serous cystadenomas and pancreatic neuroendocrine tumors (Pancreatic NET). Cysts and Cystadenomas generally do not require treatment. Pancreatic NET should be rated on size, behavior, and DNA type. Tumors greater than 3 cm, or with a doubling rate of fewer than 500 days, should be considered for surgery. In patients with an alteration in exon 3, tumors greater than 2 cm should be considered for surgery. (Blansfield et al., *Surgery,* 2007) (See Table 1.)

References:

General:
Maher ER, Neumann HP, Richard S., von Hippel-Lindau disease: a clinical and scientific review. *Eur J Hum Genet.* 2011 Jun;19(6):617-23. Epub 2011 Mar 9. PMID: 21386872

Lonser RR, Glenn GM, Chew EY, Libutti SK, Linehan WM, Oldfield EH, von Hippel-Lindau disease. *Lancet.* 2003 Jun 14;361(9374):2059-67. PMID: 12814730

See additional articles cited in topic sections for each organ system.

Preparing for Pheo Testing

It is most important to test for pheochromocytomas before undergoing surgery for any reason, and before going through the childbirthing process. Undergoing either of these stressful experiences with an unknown pheo can be extremely dangerous. If the doctors are aware that the pheo is there, they can take preventive action that will ensure the safety of the patient, and any unborn child.

Testing of blood and urine are the best tests to determine whether an active pheo is present and whether additional scanning is needed to *localize* or find the tumor. The urine and blood tests for pheo are most reliable when care is taken in two areas—diet prior to the testing and preservation of the urine sample from the start of the test until the lab processing is complete.

To get the best information from a 24-hour urine test, it is critically important that the patient follow carefully the pheo test instructions that go with the test. Not all hospitals provide these instructions to the patient, and not all patients follow them conscientiously. Differences in instructions may reflect different methods of analysis.

If your own hospital lab staff has provided instructions, that's great! If not, ask them if the following instructions would be good to follow to ensure that the sample is fresh and that the chemical levels for which they are testing are not artificially influenced by things in your diet. It is also very important that the urine be carefully refrigerated and preserved throughout the 24-hour urine collection period and delivered fresh to the lab for immediate processing. Some people carry the jug in an insulated bag or backpack, with one or more plastic cold packs alongside the jug.

Preparation for Blood Testing

Do not take any medications, including aspirin and acetaminophen, without the knowledge and agreement of the doctor ordering the test. In particular, be sure to discuss theophylline, anti-hypertensives (blood pressure medicines), methyldopa, L-dopa, or any diuretic, birth control pills, birth control patches, smoking cessation products., or any anti-depressants or other mood-altering drugs. Theophylline is found in tea and some other herbal supplements as well as medications.

Refrain from eating or drinking anything except water from 10 p.m. the evening prior to your blood test and do not take any medications the morning of the test unless specifically approved by the doctor ordering the test. If you are instructed not to take your morning medications, take them with you to the test so that you can take them right after the completion of the test.

If you smoke, you should not smoke on the day of the test. Contact your physician if you have questions regarding your diet.

The procedure usually takes about 45 minutes. It is important that you be quiet and calm for 20–30 minutes prior to the blood draw to ensure accurate results. Bring a book to read, or an electronic device with some favorite music, something you will find relaxing. You may be asked to lie quietly on a table for 20 minutes before the test begins. Lying down helps to increase the chances that the test result will be accurate.

There is published evidence that the slight pain and mental stress of the needle stick can cause a small increase in plasma catecholamines. For this reason, the original recommendation was to insert an indwelling intravenous needle, followed by a 20 minute relaxation. There is now some evidence that this might not be so important for measurements of plasma metanephrines in adults in whom the stress of the needlestick can be minimal and very short-lasting. However, in children and adults who are clearly sensitive to needle sticks and even the anticipation of the needlestick, it is recommended to continue to insist on using an indwelling intravenous needle.

Pheos in VHL-related tumors do not produce epinephrine (adrenaline) or its metabolite metanephrine. VHL-related tumors only produce norepinephrine and its metabolite, normetanephrine. Therefore, it is the value for plasma normetanephrine that one must watch carefully in patients screened because of VHL mutations. The chemical profiles for other genetic mutation types is different.

Upper limits for reference intervals of plasma concentrations of metanephrines in children (from samples collected lying down with an indwelling i.v.) are published (Weise, *J Clin Endocrinol Metab.*, 2002)

- For boys 5 to 18 years, the upper limit for normetanephrine is 97 pg/mL (0.53 nmol/L) and for metanephrine 102 pg/mL (0.52 nmol/L).
- For girls 5 to 18 years, the upper limit for normetanephrine is 77 pg/mL (0.42 nmol/L) and for metanephrine 68 pg/mL (0.37 nmol/L).

The reference intervals for your lab may be slightly different due to variations in processing. If there are concerns about interactions with medications, it is important that the laboratory use LC-MS/MS techniques to analyze the sample, to achieve the highest sensitivity and selectivity in checking fractionated metanephrines, especially normetanephrine. (LCMS/MS stands for multidimensional chromatography coupled with mass spectometry.)

Preparation for 24-hour Urine Testing

Vanillyl Mandelic Acid testing (VMA): This test is no longer used as it does not measure fractionated metanephrines.

For Catecholamines, Metanephrines, Epinephrine, Norepinephrine: Avoid smoking, medications, chocolate, fruits (especially bananas), and caffeine on the day of the test. Be sure to tell your doctor and the technician what medications you are taking, including any anti-depressants.

Collection instructions: Do not begin collection on Friday or Saturday. This ensures that your sample will be delivered to the lab on a working day and can be processed promptly.

1. Start the collection in the morning. Empty the bladder and do not save this urine specimen.

2. Write this date and time on the jug.*
3. Save all the urine passed for the next 24 hours in the jug provided, include the final specimen passed exactly 24 hours after beginning the collection.
4. Keep the urine refrigerated at all times. You might keep it in a paper bag in the refrigerator. If you must be out, you could carry it in a bag or backpack with plastic ice packs against the jug.
5. Write this date and time on the jug when the collection is finished.
6. Bring the collection and the paper work to the lab as soon as possible after collection. (Drop it off on the way to school or work. Labs are usually open early in the morning or have a place where you can arrange to drop it off early).

* If there is a preservative added to the jug, be careful not to get it on the skin. If this happens, wash the area immediately with water.

References:

Grouzmann E, et al., Diagnostic accuracy of free and total metanephrines in plasma and fractionated metanephrines in urine of patients with pheochromocytoma, *Eur J Endocrinol.* 2010 May;162(5):951-60. Epub 2010 Feb 8. PMID: 20142367

Eisenhofer G, et al., Measurements of plasma methoxytyramine, normetanephrine, and metanephrine as disriminators of different hereditary forms of pheochromocytoma, *Clin Chem.* 2011 Mar;57(3):411-20. Epub 2011 Jan 24. PMID: 21262951

Weise M, Merke DP, Pacak K, Walther MM, Eisenhofer G. Utility of plasma free metanephrines for detecting childhood pheochromocytoma. *J Clin Endocrinol Metab.* 2002 May;87(5):1955-60. PMID: 11994324

Section 6:
Obtaining DNA Testing

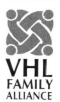

Anyone with a first- or second-degree relative with VHL is "at risk" for VHL. First degree relatives are parents, children, sisters, and brothers. Second-degree relatives are cousins, aunts, uncles, grandparents, and grandchildren of a person with VHL. Each child of a person with VHL is at 50% risk for VHL. The only way to determine for sure whether someone has VHL is through DNA testing. This is a blood test that must be processed at a clinical testing laboratory (lab) that has the necessary equipment and reagents to test for VHL, and has been certified as compliant with the Clinical Laboratory Improvement Amendments (CLIA) in the United States, or has achieved equivalent quality ratings in other countries.

If DNA testing finds the altered VHL gene, the results are positive: yes, this person has VHL. If the DNA testing finds that both copies of the VHL gene are unaltered, the test is negative: this person is unlikely to have VHL. There is always some margin for error. In a CLIA-certified lab, the possibility of error is under 1–2%, which is considered to be as certain as it gets in nature. Anyone at risk for VHL who has not received a negative DNA test result should continue to follow a conscientious screening program to ensure early diagnosis of any VHL problems.

To initiate DNA testing in a family, a person in the family with a clinical diagnosis of VHL, working through a geneticist or genetic counselor, should submit a blood sample for testing. The lab will check to see that they can determine the alteration in this person by performing a complete screen of the VHL gene, sometimes including some additional testing to look for larger deletions. Properly done, this test is greater than 99% successful in finding mutations in patients with a *germline* mutation in the VHL gene. Once a mutation has been found, the exact change in this person's VHL gene will be the same alteration that is passed within this family. Now another person in the same family who does not have a clinical diagnosis of VHL can submit a blood sample, and the lab can check for that same mutation in this second person's DNA. This first test in the family becomes a road map for subsequent tests in that family.

People who were tested prior to the year 2000 using a method called "linkage analysis" may wish to be re-tested using DNA sequencing, or more modern methods, which are significantly more reliable. There have been situations where the results of linkage analysis have proven not to be correct.

For people who are the first in their families to be diagnosed with VHL, or for adoptees or others who do not have known blood relatives to assist in the testing, it can take a little longer and cost a little more to get results from a complete screen. For people in this situation, it is important to choose a lab with experience with research teams studying VHL, that can provide a more thorough report.

It is important to initiate DNA testing through a geneticist or genetic counselor, to ensure a thorough discussion of the personal impact of the results, whether they are positive or negative, and the possible insurance ramifications. To find a geneticist or genetic counselor, check the genetic counselors' website, http://www.nsgc.org. You can search by institution, country, or postal code. Large medical centers will usually have a department of "cancer genetics." If so, this is the best place to assess your risk for VHL.

If a mother-to-be is having any genetic testing done, she may request a VHL test be part of that scope of tests, especially if there is any VHL in the family at all, or any history of VHL-related tumors in other family members.

The list of clinical testing labs offering complete testing for VHL (including large deletions) is maintained on the internet at http://genetests.org. The list of DNA testing labs with close relationships with research teams is maintained by the VHLFA at http://vhl.org/dna.

If your DNA diagnosis is unclear, please contact the VHL Family Alliance to discuss it further and to consider participating in a study to understand these situations. Contact info@vhl.org.

References:

The American Society of Human Genetics (ASHG) has information on policy and ethics on their website. See http://genetics.faseb.org/genetics/ashg/ashgmenu.htm

Collins, Debra, Information for Genetic Professionals http://www.kumc.edu/gec/prof/kugenes.html

National Library of Medicine has a list of labs that meet the standards set by CLIA
http://www.ncbi.nlm.nih.gov/sites/GeneTests/lab

National Society of Genetic Counselors has a website where you can find a genetic counselor near you. http://nsgc.org

The US government offers a tool for preparing a Family Health History document to help you and your family assess their health risks and learn to manage them.
http://familyhistory.hhs.gov

The Office of Biotechnology Activities maintains a website that contains information on the work of the Advisory Committee to the Secretary of Health and Human Services on "Genetic Testing." http://www4.od.nih.gov/oba/

The Human Genome Institute has a section on Policy and Ethics that deals with the Ethical, Legal, and Social Implications of the Human Genome Project and genetic testing
See http://www.genome.gov/PolicyEthics

Section 7:
Medical Terms

ADRENAL GLANDS (ad-REE-nal): a pair of glands on top of the kidneys which normally produce epinephrine (adrenaline) when we are stressed or excited.

ADRENALECTOMY (ad-REE-nal-EK-to-mee): surgical removal of an adrenal gland. May be partial or total.

ADRENALINE (a-DREN-a-lin) or epinephrine: A hormone secreted by the adrenal medulla upon stimulation by the central nervous system in response to stress such as anger or fear. It acts to increase heart rate, blood pressure, cardiac output and carbohydrate metabolism.

ALLELE (a-LEEL): One of the two copies of each gene in an individual. In people with VHL, one copy of the VHL gene is altered and one has the normal sequence.

ANGIOGRAM (ANN-gee-o-GRAM): A picture or map of the blood vessels in a particular area of the body, usually produced by injecting a special dye into the blood vessels and taking x-ray or magnetic resonance pictures. See also Fluorescein angiogram.

ANGIOMA (ann-gee-O-ma): An unusual growth made up of blood or lymphatic vessels, forming a benign tumor; a hemangioma (blood vessels) or lymphangioma (lymphatic vessels). In VHL, angiomas are made up of blood vessels and so are technically hemangiomas.

ANGIOMATOSIS: Another name for von Hippel-Lindau.

ASYMPTOMATIC: The patient is not experiencing discomfort or other symptoms.

AUDIOLOGY (aw-dee-OL-o-gy): The study of hearing. Often refers to a hearing test (audiogram), which determines hearing loss.

AUDIOMETRIC (aw-dee-oh-MET-rik): An audiometric examination is an examination in which the hearing is measured and evaluated.

AUTOSOME: A non sex-determining chromosome. An autosomal dominant trait is one which occurs on one of the chromosomes which do not determine gender, and is dominant because it takes only one altered copy of the gene to cause the trait.

BENIGN TUMOR (bee-NINE): An abnormal growth that is not cancer and does not spread to other parts of the body. Benign does not mean harmless, only that it does not spread.

BIOMARKER: Some trace chemical in the blood or urine that we can test for, that will indicate the progress of a disease. For example, the PSA test for prostate cancer indicates whether the prostate gland is enlarging so that you know whether you need additional testing and treatment.

BROAD LIGAMENT: The broad ligament is a folded sheet of tissue that drapes over the uterus, fallopian tubes and the ovaries.

CAPILLARIES (CAP-a-lar-reez): The smallest of the blood vessels in the body, carrying nourishment to the cells.

CANCER: A general term for more than 100 diseases in which abnormal cells grow and multiply rapidly. Cancer cells can spread through the blood or lymphatic system to start new cancers in other parts of the body.

CATECHOLAMINES (kat-e-COAL-a-meens): adrenaline by-products found in the urine or blood, where their measurement is used as a test for pheochromocytoma. Most important for VHL, is measurement of fractionated metanephrines, especially normetanephrine.

CEREBELLUM (ser-a-BELL-um): A large portion of the base of the brain which serves to coordinate voluntary movements, posture, and balance.

CEREBRAL (ser-EE-bral): The upper or main portion of the brain, often used to refer to the entire brain.

CHROMOSOME (KRO-mo-sohm): Sets of linear DNA from which the genes are arranged, carrying all the instructions for the species. Human beings have 23 pairs of chromosomes. In each pair, one chromosome, containing one copy of each gene, is inherited from the mother and one from the father.

CODON (KO-don): a triplet of three bases in a DNA molecule, a code for making a single amino acid of a protein.

COMPUTED TOMOGRAPHY (CT) scan: A diagnostic procedure using a combination of *X-ray* and computer, and optionally some contrast dye. A series of X-ray pictures are taken of the tissues being studied. The computer is then used to calculate the size and density of any tumors seen on the pictures.

CRYOTHERAPY: A method of stunting the growth of tissues by freezing them. Used most commonly on retinal angiomas.

CYSTS: Fluid-filled sacs that may occur normally in tissues from time to time, or that may grow up around irritations in tissues.

DE NOVO (day-NO-vo): New, for the first time.

DENSITY: a quality of a tissue to be soft or solid. Muscle is less dense than bone; a sac filled with fluid is less dense than a hard tumor.

DIFFERENTIAL DIAGNOSIS: Many of the tumors of VHL occur in the general population, or in other syndromes as well. The doctor has to sort out whether the tumor is *sporadic* or whether it is part of VHL or another syndrome. To answer this question a number of tests may be required, which may include DNA testing.

DNA: Deoxyribonucleic acid (DEE-ox-ee-RYE-bo-nu-KLAY-ik ASS-id). Four substances which makes up chromosomes and their genes. As coding sequences they determine the function of a gene—for instance the synthesis of a protein and the amino acid sequence of the protein.

-ECTOMY (EK-to-mee): a suffix which means removal. For example, adrenalectomy means removal of the adrenal gland.

EMBRYOLOGICAL (em-bree-o-LODGE-i-kal): Having to do with the process of development of the baby before birth. The baby starts out as a single cell, from which all organs and tissues develop. As the embryo forms, the cells evolve. The epididymis in men and the broad ligament structures in women develop from the same cells.

ENDOCRINOLOGIST (EN-do-krin-OL-o-gist): A physician specializing in the treatment of the endocrine system, its hormones, and glands, which includes the adrenal glands, pancreas and a number of other organs and glands.

ENDOLYMPHATIC SAC (en-do-lim-FA-tik sack): the bulb-like end of the endolymphatic duct, which connects to the semicircular canals of the inner ear.

ENUCLEATION (ee-NU-klee-A-shun): *Referring to kidney or pancreas,* removal of a tumor with only a small margin of healthy tissue to ensure that all the unhealthy tissue is out. This is sometimes referred to as a lumpectomy, or removal of the tumor (lump) only. *In ophthalmology,* enucleation means removal of the eye. If the retina has detached, the blood supply to the eye is reduced and the eye may deteriorate, causing discomfort. If this occurs, enucleation of the eye may be recommended. A good prosthesis (artificial eyeball), can be made to look like a healthy eye.

EPIDIDYMIS (epi-DID-imus): A gland which lies behind the testicle, in the scrotum, on the path to the vas deferens, the vessel that carries the sperm from the testicle to the prostate gland, and is important for sperm maturation, mobility and storage.

EPINEPHRINE (eh-pin-EFF-rin): See ADRENALINE.

FALLOPIAN TUBE (fa-LOPE-i-an): the channel carrying eggs from the ovary to the uterus.

FAMILIAL (fam-EE-lee-al): It occurs in families, whether or not transmitted genetically. Chicken pox is considered familial, but is not genetic.

FLUORESCEIN ANGIOGRAM (FLUR-a-seen AN-gio-gram): An angiogram of the retina of the eye, named for the contrast dye that is used. This procedure produces an image of the blood vessels of the retina, sometimes in full motion video so that the ophthalmologist can see the health of the blood vessels and how the blood moves through them.

GADOLINIUM (gad-o-LIN-ee-um): a contrast medium, injected into the patient's bloodstream prior to an MRI test to highlight the blood vessels and provide better contrast so the radiologist can see any abnormal structures more clearly.

GASTROENTEROLOGIST (GAS-tro-en-ter-OL-o-jist): A physician who specializes in the diagnosis and treatment of disorders of the gastrointestinal tract, including the esophagus, stomach, small intestine, pancreas, liver, gall bladder, and biliary system (liver).

GENE (jeen): The position on a chromosome where a specific DNA sequence, or allele, resides. Changes in the sequence from one allele to another can be transmitted to the next generation.

GENETIC COUNSELOR: A medical professional (not a physician) specializing in working with patients and families with genetically inherited conditions like VHL. Genetic counseling may include a discussion and analysis of your family tree and some testing procedures.

GENETICIST: A geneticist is a scientist specializing in the study of genes and the way they influence our health, and in treatment of genetic disorders.

GENOME (JEE-nohm): The entire array of genes of an organism or species.

GENOTYPE (JEE-no-type): The particular pair of alleles (copies of the gene) that an individual possesses at a given gene locus or site (two copies of each gene). One of these alleles (copies) is inherited from the mother, the other from the father. The genotype describes the configuration of the altered gene.

GERMLINE (JERM-line): any genetic alteration that occurs in every cell of the body, including testes in men and the ovaries in women, that produce the sperm and eggs that will become children.

-GRAM: a suffix that indicates that a message or picture is being created. For example, an angiogram is a picture of the blood vessels (ANGIO-).

HEMANGIOMA (hee-MAN-jee-O-ma): An abnormal growth of blood vessels, forming a benign tumor.

HEMANGIOBLASTOMA (hee-MAN-jee-o-blast-O-ma): An abnormal growth of blood vessels forming a benign tumor; a variety of hemangioma found especially in VHL, in the brain or spinal cord.

HEREDITARY: Occurring because of something in the genes you got from your parents, something you inherited. Not due to infection or an event during your lifetime.

HYPERNEPHROMA (hyper-nef-ROH-ma): A kidney tumor that contains cancer cells. The more modern term is renal cell carcinoma (RCC).

INVASIVE: Describes medical procedures that require entering or "invading" your body.

KIDNEY: One of a pair of organs in back of the abdominal cavity that filter waste materials out of the blood and pass them out of the body as urine.

LAPAROSCOPY (lap-ar-OSS-ko-pee): A technique for performing a surgical procedure through slits in the skin using special surgical probes, rather than making one large incision. Depending on the position of the tumor and the extensiveness of the procedure, use of this technique may or may not be possible.

LASER TREATMENT: The surgical use of a minutely focused light to deliver a microscopic cauterization, or burn.

LESION: Any localized abnormal structural change, such as an ANGIOMA.

LIVER: A large organ in the upper right side of the abdominal cavity that secretes bile and is active in regulating various parts of the process of digesting food and using it to best advantage in the body.

LOCALIZE: To find. Doctors use this term to mean finding on the scan exactly where a tumor is located. For a pheo, for example, the tumor can occur anywhere from your groin to your earlobe, on either side of the body, so finding a pheo is not an easy quest.

MAGNETIC RESONANCE IMAGING (MRI). An imaging technique where magnetic energy is used to examine tissues in your body, and the information is used by a computer to create an image. There is no radiation exposure. The resulting images look very much like *X-rays*, but include images of soft tissues (like blood vessels) as well as hard tissues (like bones). Claustrophobia can be an issue, since this procedure requires lying still in a tunnel-like structure for at least half an hour. Calming drugs can be used, or there are new machines that have a more open, cage-like structure, and various attempts are being made to shorten the time required. It is important to use enough magnet strength to get a clear picture.

MALIGNANT (ma-LIG-nant): Cancerous. Cancer cells can spread through the blood or lymphatic system to start new cancers in other parts of the body.

METANEPHRINES (met-a-NEF-rins): a group of adrenaline by-products found in the urine or blood, where its measurement is used as a test for pheochromocytoma. Fractionated metanephrines assay breaks the group of metanephrines into its component parts (metanephrine and normetanephrine) and measures them separately. It is the measure of normetanephrine which is the most accurate indicator of pheo in VHL. Calculations differ for other pheo syndromes.

METASTASIZE (me-TAS-ta-size): to spread from one part of the body to another. When cancer cells metastasize and form secondary tumors, the cells in the metastatic tumor are like those in the original tumor. Thus if kidney cancer cells are found in a tumor in the spine, we know it has metastasized, or spread, from the kidney.

MIBG SCAN: A nuclear medicine procedure using a radioactive isotope or tracer, which is absorbed by pheochromocytoma tissue. Meta-Iodo-Benzyl-Guanidine (MIBG) is injected into the patient before the scan is performed, making the pheo stand out clearly on the diagnostic pictures.

MLPA or Multiplex Ligation-Dependent Probe Amplification is a newer, more efficient, and more accurate procedure for analyzing a DNA sample.

MONITORING: Monitoring is checking up on known issues, to make sure that they are treated at the best time to insure long-term health. You and your medical team will work out the right interval for checkups, depending on your particular situation.

MUTATION: A change in the sequence of DNA coding in a gene.

MYELOGRAM (MY-lo-GRAM): a diagnostic procedure which creates an image of the spinal cord. A dye is injected into the spinal canal, and X-ray pictures are taken of the spinal cord.

NEOPLASIA (NEE-oh-PLAY-zia): literally, new growth, a lesion grown from a single cell, not transplanted from another place.

NEPHRECTOMY (nef-REK-to-mee): Removal of all (total) or some (partial) of one kidney.

NEUROENDOCRINE (NEW-ro-EN-do-krin) Having to do with the interactions between the nervous system and the endocrine system, which secretes (produces) hormones. Neuroendocrine describes certain cells that release hormones (neurohormone) into the blood in response to stimulation of the nervous system. In VHL these are found in pheochromocytomas and pancreatic neuroendocrine tumors.

NEUROLOGIST: A physician specializing in nonsurgical treatment of the nervous system, the brain, spinal cord and peripheral nerves.

NEUROSURGEON: A physician specializing in the surgical treatment of the nervous system, the brain, spinal cord, and peripheral nerves.

NEUROTOLOGIST (new-ro-TOLL-uh-jist): A physician specializing in the structure and function of the internal ear, its neural connections with the brain and the management of skull base diseases. A neurotologist is an ear, nose and throat surgeon (otolaryngologist) who has undergone additional training in this area and typically works in conjunction with a team of specialists including other otolaryngologists, neurologists and neurosurgeons.

NORADRENALINE (NOR-a-DREN-a-lin): The metabolite of adrenaline, produced when adrenaline is metabolized or processed by the body.

NOREPINEPHRINE (see NORADRENALINE)

NORMETANEPHRINE (NOR-meta-NEF-rin): The metabolite of metanephrine, produced when metanephrine is broken down by the body.

NUCLEAR MEDICINE: Medical procedures for diagnosis and treatment which involve some sort of radioactive isotope.

ONCOLOGIST (on-KOL-o-gist): A physician specializing in treatment of various forms of cancer.

OPHTHALMOLOGIST (OFF-thal-MOL-o-gist): A physician specializing in treatment of diseases of the eye.

OPTOMETRIST (op-TOM-e-trist): An optometrist, or doctor of optometry (O.D.) is a health care professional who diagnoses and treats eye health and vision problems.

They prescribe glasses, contact lenses, low vision rehabilitation, vision therapy and medications, and perform some surgical procedures not related to VHL.

PANCREAS (PAN-kree-as): A gland near the stomach which secretes digestive enzymes into the intestine and also secretes the hormone insulin into the blood as needed to regulate the level of sugar in the blood.

Pancreatic NET: Pancreatic Neuro-endocrine Tumor, a solid tumor of the islet-cell portion of the pancreas which secretes hormones when it is "active". The abbreviation PNET is also used to refer to two other tumors which are not related to VHL.

PANCREATITIS (pan-kree-a-TIE-tis): inflammation of the pancreas.

PAPILLARY (PAP-i-lar-ry): nipple-shaped.

PARAGANGLIOMA (PAR-a-GAN-glee-OH-ma): A pheo outside of the adrenal gland, which is also called an extra-adrenal pheochromocytoma (extra meaning "outside"). In this book they are referred to as pheos. Paraganglioma is the term most frequently applied to pheos of the head and neck.

PENETRANCE: The probability that a gene will make any effect of its alteration evident. The VHL gene has almost complete penetrance (if someone has the altered VHL gene, they will almost certainly have some manifestation of VHL disease within their lifetime), but widely variable expression (the severity of those manifestations will vary widely).

PET SCANNING: Positron Emission Tomography, a specialized imaging technique using short-lived radioactive substances to provide information about the body's chemistry. This technique produces three-dimensional color images showing the activity level of certain tumors.

PHENOTYPE (FEE-no-type): The clinical appearance of a specific genotype, for example the set of VHL symptoms one person may have. The same genotype may be expressed differently from one individual to the next due to differences in other genes, or in the environment.

PHEOCHROMOCYTOMA (FEE-o-KRO-mo-sigh-TOE-mah): or "pheo" for short. A tumor (cytoma) of the adrenal gland which causes the adrenal gland to secrete too much adrenalin, potentially causing harm to the heart and blood vessels. Pheos can also occur outside the adrenal glands, and people can have more than two pheos. Outside the adrenals, they are sometimes called paragangliomas.

PNET or Pancreatic NET: Pancreatic Neuro-endocrine Tumor, a solid tumor of the islet-cell portion of the pancreas which secretes hormones when it is "active". The abbreviation PNET is also used to refer to two other tumors which are not related to VHL.

PMID: An abbreviation for PubMed ID, the catalog number for an article catalogued in an internet resource, http://www.pubmed.com. To find "PMID: 18799446" go to PubMed and search for 18799446. The catalog will display the abstract of the article, and will tell you how to obtain the full text in English and sometimes also in additional languages.

RADIO FREQUENCY ABLATION (RFA): A laparoscopic surgical procedure where a heat probe is inserted laparoscopically into the tumor, and the tumor is heated to disable its growth potential. This is one possible way to treat a VHL kidney tumor.

RADIOLOGIST: A physician specializing in diagnostic techniques for viewing internal organs and tissues without surgery. Radiological methods include X-ray, MRI, computed tomography (CT) scan, ultrasound, angiography, and nuclear isotopes.

RENAL CELL CARCINOMA (RCC): Cancer of the kidney.

RESECTION (ree-SEK-shun): A term used to describe the removal of a tumor from an organ such as a kidney, while retaining (sparing) the organ itself.

RETINA: The nerve tissue that lives at the back of the eye, similar to the film in a camera, which takes the image you are looking at and transmits it to the brain through the optic nerve. This area is nourished by a web of very fine blood vessels.

RETINAL SPECIALIST: An ophthalmologist who specializes in treatment of diseases of the retina.

SCREENING: Testing before symptoms appear, to make sure that any issues are found early. It is best not to wait for symptoms.

SEROUS MICROCYSTIC ADENOMAS: Grapelike clusters of cysts which may occur in the pancreas. Cysts are composed of epithelium-lined collections of serous fluid that vary in size from several millimeters to over 10 cm. (over four inches).

SIGN: Physical evidence of the existence of something which can be demonstrated by a medical doctor.

SPORADIC: Occurring at random in the general population. Not due to heredity.

SYMPATHETIC NERVOUS SYSTEM: a chain of small structures that transmit signals from the central nervous system to the organs. The adrenal gland is the major gland in this chain, but small ganglia run from the groin to the ear lobe on both sides of the body. A pheochromocytoma can hide anywhere along this system.

SYMPTOM: A feeling or other subjective complaint suggestive of a medical condition.

SYMPTOMATIC: The patient is experiencing symptoms.

SYNDROME: A collection of signs and symptoms associated with a disease.

SYRINX (SEER-inks): A fluid-filled sac, like a cyst, but occurring inside the spine where it has the shape of an elongated tube lying along or inside the spinal cord and inside the bony spinal column.

TINNITUS (TIN-ih-tis): A ringing in one or both ears. It may also be a roaring or hissing sound.

TUMOR: An abnormal growth that is solid and may be benign or malignant.

ULTRASOUND: A diagnostic technique that provides pictures of internal organs and structures. It works like the sonar used by submarines, bouncing sound waves off an object and using a computer to interpret the sound returned. The interpretation of an ultrasound is very dependent upon body structure, the amount of body fat, and the skill of the operator.

UROLOGIST: A physician specializing in surgical and non-surgical treatment of the kidney, bladder and male genital organs, including the penis and scrotal structures.

VERTIGO (VER-tih-go): A sensation of dizziness or loss of balance, inability to walk a straight line, or "walking into walls".

VISCERA (VISS-ser-ah): Any of a number of organs in the abdominal area, including the kidney, liver, pancreas, and adrenal glands.

X-RAY: A diagnostic imaging technique where radiation passes through the body to create images of hard tissues (like bones and solid tumors) onto photographic film.

Section 8:
Prepared by

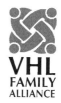

This original International English edition was prepared by Members of the VHL Family Alliance
— *Edited by Joyce Wilcox Graff*

with the kind assistance of
Lloyd M. Aiello, M.D., Beetham Eye Institute, Joslin Diabetes Center, Boston, Massachusetts
Lloyd P. Aiello, M.D., Ph.D., Beetham Eye Institute, Joslin Diabetes Center, Boston, Massachusetts
Marie Luise Bisgaard, Institute for Molecular Medicine, University of Copenhagen, Denmark
Gennady Bratslavsky, M.D., Urology, State University of New York Upstate Medical University, Syracuse, New York
Michael Brown, O.D., Veterans Administration, Huntsville, Alabama
Jerry D. Cavallerano, Ph.D., Optometry, Joslin Diabetes Center, Boston, Massachusetts
Emily Y. Chew, M.D., Ophthalmology, National Eye Institute, Bethesda, Maryland
Daniel Choo, M.D., Otolaryngology, Children's Hospital Medical Center, Cincinnati, Ohio
Debra L. Collins, M.S., Department of Genetics, University of Kansas Medical Center, Kansas City
Maria Czyzyk-Krzeska, Ph.D., Vontz Center for Molecular Studies, University of Cincinnati Medical Center, Cincinnati, Ohio
Molly Daniels, M.S., C.G.C., Clinical Cancer Genetics, M.D. Anderson Cancer Center, Houston, Texas
Jochen Decker, M.D., Ph.D., Oncology, Johannes Gutenberg University of Mainz, Germany
Graeme Eisenhofer, Ph.D., Neurochemistry, University of Dresden, Germany
Yasser El-Sayed, M.D., Obstetrics, Stanford University Medical Center, Palo Alto, California

Joal Fischer, M.D. and Tina B. Farney, SupportWorks, Charlotte, North Carolina

Rachel Giles, Ph.D., Nephrology, University Medical Center, Utrecht, The Netherlands, and President of the Dutch VHL Family Alliance

Vincent Giovannucci, O.D., medical cartoonist, Auburn, Massachusetts

Gladys M. Glenn, M.D., Ph.D., Cancer Epidemiology and Genetics, National Institutes of Health, Bethesda, Maryland

James Gnarra, Ph.D., Urology and Pathology, University of Pittsburgh, Pittsburgh, Pennsylvania

Michael B. Gorin, M.D., Ophthalmology, University of Southern California, Los Angeles, California

Jane Green, M.S., Ph.D., Community Medicine, Health Sciences Center, St. John's, Newfoundland, Canada

David J. Gross, M.D., Endocrinology, Hadassah-Hebrew University Medical Center, Jerusalem, Israel

Tina Gruner, R.D., C.D.E., Mountain View Medical Associates, Madras, Oregon

Pascal Hammel, M.D., Gastroenterology, Hôpital Beaujon, Clichy, France

Adrian Harris, M.D., Ph.D., Cancer Research, Churchill Hospital, Oxford, England, UK

Yujen Edward Hsia, M.D., Medical Genetics, Retired, Honolulu, Hawaii

Tien Hsu, Ph.D., Hematology and Medical Oncology, Boston University School of Medicine, Boston, Massachusetts

Howard Hughes Medical Institute, Chevy Chase, Maryland

Othon Iliopoulos, M.D., Familial Renal Cell Cancer Program, Massachusetts General Hospital, Boston, Massachusetts

G. P. James, M.S., Medical writer, and Frank James, Illustrator, Springfield, Ohio

Eric Jonasch, M.D., Urologic Oncology, M.D. Anderson Cancer Center, Houston, Texas

William G. Kaelin, Jr., Genetics, Dana-Farber Cancer Institute, Boston, Massachusetts

Jeffrey Kim, M.D., Neurotology, Georgetown University Medical Center, Washington, D.C., and National Institute of Neurological Disorders and Stroke, Bethesda, Maryland

James M. Lamiell, M.D., Clinical Investigation Regulatory Office, Retired, Fort Sam Houston, Texas

Jacques W. M. Lenders, M.D., Internal Medicine, St. Radboud University Hospital, Nymegen, the Netherlands

Richard Alan Lewis, M.D., M.S., Ophthalmology, Pediatrics and Genetics, Cullen Eye Institute, Baylor College of Medicine, Houston, Texas

John Libertino, M.D., Urology, Lahey Clinic, Burlington, Massachusetts

Steven K. Libutti, M.D., Director, Einstein-Montefiore Center for Cancer Care, New York, New York

W. Marston Linehan, Chief, Urologic Oncology, National Cancer Institute, Bethesda, Maryland

Cornelius J. M. Lips, M.D., Retired, University Hospital, Utrecht, the Netherlands.

Joseph A. Locala, M.D., Psychiatry and Psychology, Cleveland Clinic Foundation, Cleveland, Ohio

Russell R. Lonser, M.D., Surgical Neurology Branch, National Institute of Neurological Disorders and Stroke, Bethesda, Maryland

Eamonn R. Maher, M.D., Medical Genetics, University of Birmingham, Birmingham, England, U.K.

Patrick Maxwell, M.D., Ph.D., Nephrology, University College London, England, UK

Ian McCutcheon, M.D., FRCSC, Neurosurgery, M.D. Anderson Cancer Center, Houston, Texas

Scott McLean, M.D., Genetics, San Antonio Genetics, San Antonio, Texas

Virginia V. Michels, M.D., Medical Genetics, Mayo Clinic, Rochester, Minnesota

Alessandra Murgia M.D. Ph.D., Pediatrics and Genetics, University of Padua, Italy

Haring J.W. Nauta, M.D., Ph.D., Neurosurgery, Retired, University of Texas, Galveston, Texas

Hartmut P. H. Neumann, M.D., Department of Nephrology, Albert-Ludwigs University, Freiburg, Germany, and the VHL Study Group in Germany

Edward H. Oldfield, M.D., Surgical Neurology, University of Virginia, Charlottesville, Virginia

Karel Pacak, M.D., Ph.D., DSc, Medical Neuroendocrinology, National Institute of Child Health and Human

Development, National Institutes of Health, Bethesda, Maryland

Stephen Pautler, M.D., FRCS, Urology, St. Joseph's Hospital, London, Ontario

Arnim Pause, Ph.D., Biochemistry, McGill University, Montreal, Quebec, Canada

Marie Louise Mølgaard Poulsen, International Health, Immunology and Microbiology, University of Copenhagen, Denmark

Stéphane Richard, M.D., Ph.D., Oncogenetics, Faculté de Médecine, Paris-Sud and Bicêtre Hospital, Le Kremlin-Bicêtre, France, and the International French-Speaking VHL Study Group

Armand Rodriguez, M.D., Internal Medicine, Fort Lauderdale, Florida

R. Neil Schimke, M.D., Ph.D., Endocrinology and Genetics, University of Kansas Medical Center, Kansas City, Kansas

Laura Schmidt, Ph.D., Urologic Oncology, National Cancer Institute, National Institutes of Health, Bethesda, Maryland

Taro Shuin, M.D., Urology, Kochi Medical School, Kochi, Japan

Cecile Skrzynia, M.S., C.G.C., Director of Cancer Genetic Counseling Services, University of North Carolina, Chapel Hill

Philippe E. Spiess, M.D., M.S., FACS, FRCS, Genitourinary Oncology, Moffitt Cancer Center, Tampa, Florida

The Illustration Studios of Stansbury, Ronsaville, Wood

Karina Villar Gómez de las Heras, M.D., President of La Alianza de las Familias VHL, Ministry of Health and Social Welfare for Castilla-LaMancha, Toledo, Spain

Steven G. Waguespack, M.D., FAAP, FACE, Endocrine Neoplasia & Hormonal Disorders, University of Texas M.D. Anderson Cancer Center, Houston, Texas

Robert B. Welch, M.D., Emeritus Professor of Ophthalmology, Johns Hopkins University School of Medicine and Greater Baltimore Medical Center, Baltimore, Maryland

Gary L. Wood, Psy.D., Psychology, Wood and Associates, Tampa, Florida

Berton Zbar, M.D., Laboratory of Immunobiology, Retired, National Cancer Institute, Frederick Cancer Research and Development Center, Frederick, Maryland

Section 9:
Tissue Bank
Your Contribution to VHL Research

We are constantly striving to increase the level of VHL research. Once considered only "an obscure medical curiosity", VHL is becoming one of the most important diseases in the study of cancer. It is the leading hereditary cause of kidney cancer. Even in cases of sporadic kidney cancer in the general population, damage that may occur to the VHL gene is implicated in the advance of kidney and other cancers. While it is estimated that only one person in 32,000 has VHL, it is estimated that 60,000 people a year in the United States alone will develop kidney cancer each year, of which 75% are clear cell renal cell carcinoma, 90% of whom will have changes in the VHL gene in their tumors — altogether 40,500 people each year with VHL-negative clear cell renal cell carcinoma, for whom we need the same drugs and therapies we need to cure VHL.

VHL is also the leading cause of genetic pheochromocytoma, accounting for approximately 30% of all pheos. Again, studying VHL and the six other genetic causes of pheos is giving us a much keener appreciation of the genetic pathway, or chain of events, that can lead to a pheo, or which conversely might provide clues on how to cure them.

As the level of VHL research increases, the need for VHL tissue for research also increases. It is here that we can help. The VHL Family Alliance established a VHL Tissue Bank in 1995. We are working to enhance our banking to make this an even more attractive resource for researchers. Tissue donated by VHL patients is held in the Tissue Bank until an approved research project has need for it.

If you have been diagnosed with VHL, and are contemplating surgery, you can help the research community by donating any surgically removed tissue to the VHL Tissue Bank. All cost and arrangements for recovery and transfer of tissue will be taken care of by the Tissue Bank. If you would like to help the VHL research effort, please contact the tissue banking project nearest you and make arrangements to donate surgically removed tissue. All information will be treated in the strictest confidence. Pre-registration makes the process simple in the event of surgery. Simply contact the Tissue Bank, give them the name and contact information for the surgeon and the date of surgery, and the Tissue Bank will make all the necessary arrangements. Even if you are not already pre-registered, arrangements can be made by contacting the Tissue Bank.

Give a gift that only you can give, and help promote research on VHL.

Researchers interested in access to tissue on file should send requests to the Research Management Committee, VHL Family Alliance, e-mail: research@vhl.org or contact the Bank directly at bank@vhl.org

Please fill out the information requested on the forms on the following pages and mail it to the Tissue Bank for your region of the world. Contact your country support group for information, or write to info@vhl.org.

A current listing of the Tissue Banks for the various countries and regions of the world is maintained at www.vhl.org/bank. Contact info@vhl.org if your country is not listed.

Donor Registration Form
Tissue Bank for VHL Research

I, _____, wish to register myself (or a dependent minor or ward) as a VHL tissue donor with the **VHL Tissue Bank**. This donation grants permission for the **VHL Tissue Bank** to make every attempt within its means to coordinate recovery of surgically removed tissue of the above named donor. Further, if death should occur, I (**do**___ or **do not**___) hereby grant permission for recovery of brain and other tissues. All tissue is donated for the expressed purpose of furthering the research of **von Hippel-Lindau disease**.

Donor name _____

    Address _____

    City _____

    State/Province _____ Zip/Postcode _____

    Phone Day _____

    Phone Evening _____

Next of Kin _____

    Address _____

    City _____

    State/Province _____ Zip/Postcode _____

    Phone Day _____

    Phone Evening _____

Signature of Donor or Legal Guardian

    Date _____

Additional forms may be required by the Bank.

Please enclose the brief Medical/Family history on the following page, or on other paper.

Brief Medical History for the Tissue Bank

Donor's Date of Birth _____ (mm/dd/yyyy)

Sex _____ Ethnic Group _____

Has the Donor been diagnosed as having VHL? Yes___ No___

When was the diagnosis made?_____

Was a DNA test for VHL performed? _____

By whom? _____

If you (the Donor) are not diagnosed with VHL, are you the parent or relative of someone who is? Yes___ No___

Results of the DNA testing if available: _____

Age at first diagnosis: _____

Age at first symptom: _____

What were the first symptoms? _____

What relatives have VHL? _____

_____

What treatments have been performed? _____

_____

_____

_____

Feel free to include any further relevant information.

Please mail to: the **VHL Tissue Bank** for your region, found on the internet at http://www.vhl.org/bank or by contacting the VHL Family Alliance.

IMPORTANT: *In case of surgical emergency or in case of death, please notify the tissue bank **immediately** (any time, day or night). Tissue not recovered within 24 hours cannot be used for research.*

Section 10:
Keeping Current

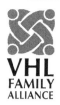

The world of medicine is changing rapidly. Working together since 1993, the VHL community — patients, physicians, and scientists — has made great strides in learning to control VHL and manage health.

In order to reach families and physicians in their native languages, a team of volunteer translators has worked hard to translate this book into a growing number of languages. For that reason, we have worked to keep this book as straightforward and stable as possible.

Once you have identified an issue in VHL, you will need the latest information on how to manage that issue — treatments will vary depending on where it is, how big it is, and a variety of other characteristics that your own medical team can help you to evaluate.

If you need assistance in finding sources of second opinions, please feel free to communicate with the VHL Family Alliance contacts in your country. A list of local support groups is maintained on the internet at vhl.org or write to info@vhl.org.

The internet is serving to help you find support even if you live in a remote area with no transportation. Please reach out to the online support resources you will find on vhl.org/support.

If you do not have access to the internet, you can still use the telephone to call 1-800-767-4VHL, toll-free in the U.S., Canada, and Mexico. Others are welcome to call, fax, or write to the addresses in this book.

Please share what you have learned, and tap into the wonderful support community of which you are now a part.

Health care professionals are welcome to call these same numbers, or to contact any of our clinical care centers of medical advisors to request input on a case.

We hope too that you will find the VHL Handbook Kids' Edition (2009) helpful in speaking with your children, whether or not they themselves have VHL. A committee of parents and professionals worked to create this book, to help you have a constructive and hopeful conversation with your children about VHL. The future for children with VHL is not like the past. People with VHL today who take an active role in maintaining their health have a better opportunity than ever before to live a full and happy life.

We hope that you will become a contributing member of the Alliance. We need all the families, friends, physicians, and researchers working together to find a cure.

The mission of the VHL Family Alliance is

TO IMPROVE DIAGNOSIS,

TREATMENT,

AND QUALITY OF LIFE FOR ALL PEOPLE AFFECTED BY VHL.

Please help achieve that goal!

Publications of the VHL Family Alliance

VHL Handbook (2012)
VHL Handbook Kids' Edition (2009)
Your Family Health Tree (2008)

Resources on the internet:

Online support groups
Online search engine
Latest information on diagnosis and treatment
See http://vhl.org

Support our Efforts!

We depend on our supporters to help fund our urgent efforts to find a cure for VHL.

Mail to:
VHLFA, 2001 Beacon St., Ste 208 Boston, MA 02135-7787 USA
or Canadian VHLFA, 4227 Hamilton Rd., Dorchester, ON N0L 1G3

Enclosed is my tax-deductible gift to support:
VHLFA: ❏ Research and Education ❏ Research only
    ❏ $25 ❏ $50 ❏ $100 ❏ $500 ❏ $1000

❏ My employer will match my donation. I have enclosed the necessary forms.

(Please make checks payable to VHL Family Alliance)

Name _____

Address _____

City _____

State/Province _____ Zip/Postcode _____

Country (if outside the U.S.) _____

Tel: _____ Fax: _____

E-mail: _____

I am a ❏ Person with VHL ❏ Family member ❏ Friend ❏ Sponsor
❏ Health professional. Specialty _____

Please charge my ❏ Mastercard ❏ Visa ❏ Amex

Card # _____ Expiration date: _____

Name as it appears on the card: _____

Signature _____

My donation is ❏ In Honor of... ❏ In Memory of... _____

Address _____

Please list the topics you would like to see addressed in future newsletters or at the Annual Meeting, and your feedback on this Handbook. Thank you!

_____
_____
_____
_____
_____
_____
_____
_____
_____
_____
_____
_____
_____

* The VHL Family Alliance is registered as a non-profit charity with the tax authorities in the United States (Tax ID# 04-3180414), Canada, and Great Britain, as well as other countries. Please contact your local group and your tax advisor for specific information on guidelines for tax deductibility of donations.

Please mail this form to VHL Family Alliance International, 2001 Beacon Street, Suite 208, Boston, MA 02135-7787 USA. *Thank you!*

VHL Family Alliance International

Jeanne W. McCoy, Chairman of the Board
Ilene Sussman, Ph.D., Executive Director

Directors:

Michelle Cieslak
Sunny Greene
Fred M. Johnson
Camron King
Robert Kramer, D.M.D.

Jane McMahon
Sarah Nielsen, M.S., C.G.C.
Thomas Rath, Ph.D.
Thomas D. Rodenberg, Esq.
Bill B. Scheitler

Council of International Affiliates:

Gerhard Alsmeier, Germany
Gilles Brunet, France
Jean-Joseph Crampe, France
Mikael Eriksson, Sweden
Carlos Alberto Fredes, Argentina
Rachel Giles, Ph.D., Netherlands
Kan Gong, M.D., P. R. China
Myriam Gorospe, Ph.D., Maryland, USA
David Gross, M.D., Israel
M. Luisa Guerra, Italy
Markus Jansen van Vuuren, South Africa
Valerie & Jon Johnson, New Zealand
Jennifer Kingston, Australia
Susan Lamb, Canada
Edith Lassus-Laurent, France
Francesco Lombardi, Italy
Jamile Mansour, Brazil
Jill Shields, Canada
M. Shinkai, Japan
Jens Strandgaard, Denmark
Helga Süli-Vargha, Ph.D., Hungary
Darko & Tamara Supuk, Croatia
Hanako Suzuki, Japan
Erika Trutmann, Switzerland
Paul & Gay Verco, Australia
Karina Villar, M.D., Spain
Michael Walker, Australia
Mary Weetman, M.S., United Kingdom
Dirk Werbrouck, Belgium

Made in the USA
Lexington, KY
02 February 2013